Water Aerobics For Seniors

Complete Guide To No-Impact Water Exercises For Seniors & Everyone Else To Help You Lose Weight And Tone Your Body

Introduction

As we start to reach our golden years, the challenges of old age begin to catch up. The body's metabolism starts to slow down, which makes losing excess body fat a real struggle, and health problems also creep in slowly.

What most people don't know is that exercises can guarantee and offset many of the ravages of time and age. The benefits you stand to gain from doing exercises are so many that they outweigh any excuses you may have for not making exercise an integral part of your daily life.

If you've been struggling with weight loss, especially in your golden years, or you are looking for ways to keep fit while having fun, then water aerobics is the answer you've been seeking.

Physical activity—of any kind—is good for your mind, soul, and body. However, with conventional exercises such as strength training, the possibility of injury or struggling to perform some exercises using the correct form is always high, especially for seniors who have brittle bones and well-worn joints. That's why most people give up a few weeks into the workout routine. Water aerobics do not have such limitations.

Besides putting less stress on your joints, water exercises and aerobics also largely eliminate the possibility of accidents and problems associated with other forms of exercise. Moreover, you don't need to be a good swimmer to engage in water aerobics: you can perform the exercises in shallow water, in an upright—standing—position.

If you would like to learn more about water aerobics, this comprehensive, easy-to-follow guide will give you everything you need to know, including the benefits and exercises you can use to get started on water aerobics.

Let's dive right into the deep end:

PS: I'd like your feedback. If you are happy with this book, please leave a review on Amazon.

Please leave a review for this book on Amazon by visiting the page below:

https://amzn.to/2VMR5qr

Table of Content

Section 1: Understanding Water Aerobics

The first thing we need to do is cultivate a deep understanding of water aerobics:

What Is Water Aerobics?

The term water aerobics refers to aerobics exercises done in water that is waist-deep or deeper water, like in a swimming pool. We can consider it a type of resistance training that focuses on aerobic endurance and comfortability.

There are different forms of water aerobics; they include water yoga, aqua Zumba, aqua jog, and aqua aerobics.

If you're wondering:

"What makes water aerobics better than other forms of exercise?"

To help answer that question, let's look at some of the most standout reasons why water aerobics are one of the best forms of exercise for seniors—and other people—who want to lose weight:

The Benefits Of Water Aerobics

The benefits of engaging in water aerobics are many because besides comfort, mainly staying cool while in a pool, the workout itself has many perks. For instance, water aerobics can help you achieve your fitness goals without breaking a sweat.

Here are other reasons why you should engage in water aerobics:

1: You can lose weight easily and quickly

One of the main advantages of engaging in water aerobics is that if you are consistent, you will lose a significant amount of body weight in a short time.

On average, just 1 hour of aerobic exercises can help you burn approximately 400 to 600 calories, a fact evident in research conducted by the Texas Research Laboratory. The research showed that every minute of water aerobics burns about ten calories. That means if you work out a minimum of 3 to 4 times a week, it will result in measurable weight loss in a short time. Worth mentioning here is that how fast and how much weight you lose will depend on how often and how much you exercise.

It takes about 3500 calories to burn one pound of fat from your body. Therefore, the more you exercise, the more calories you will burn, and, in extension, the more weight you shall lose.

When you engage in water aerobics and other exercises, your body burns more calories because it has to keep you warm. Moreover, the water massages your muscles in a way that tones them.

2: It can enhance your flexibility

As you engage in water aerobics, the water pushes and pulls your joints and muscles in unique ways. With time, your body gets used to those movements, which can lead to enhanced flexibility, allowing your joints to move in ways they previously couldn't.

Moreover, when you expose your body to the push and pull effect, it also pushes back to counter the pushing and pulling motion of the water. This constant pushing, pulling, and the overall movement is the reason why your joints become flexible in ways they weren't before. Water aerobics is like light yoga in the sense that when you stretch your muscles, they stretch and contract to adjust to the new movements.

When you subject your body to water exercises, the resistance of the water will cause your joints to increase their range of motion, thus improving your flexibility.

3: It's a low impact exercise

Another great advantage of water aerobics as a form of exercise is that, unlike other forms of exercise, it is easy on the joints.

Because of gravity, when you exercise on dry land, it exerts too much pressure on your joints, which may result in all kinds of injuries. As gravity pulls you down every time you land, it results in a significant impact shock that can have adverse effects on your physiological structure.

Typically, when you exercise in water, it causes you to become buoyant, which counteracts the forces of gravity and remove it from the equation. That means when you perform any exercise activity in a pool of water, say running, you don't exert too much pressure on your joints, which means you won't experience the same impact you would on dry land.

In essence, that means water aerobics make it possible to engage in strenuous exercises without taxing your joints, which makes water aerobics incredibly convenient if you are in your golden years and suffering from any joint problems.

In such a case, water aerobics allows you to exercise without damaging your joints further.

Additionally, water aerobics can help alleviate joint stress and relieve pain for arthritis or osteoporosis patients.

4: It can help strengthen your muscles

One of the many advantages you stand to gain from water aerobics is that the exercises will help you build muscle strength.

Sure, other exercises like strength training can help you build muscle strength too. However, unlike water aerobics, these exercises will require you to go to a gym or have special equipment. With water aerobics, all you need is a way to submerge in water: that's all.

Technically, Water aerobics is a form of resistance training. Water can add 4-42 times the amount of resistance that air produces typically. That alone makes the exercises you do in water more effective than other workouts you do outside the water.

Worth noting here is that the resistance will vary depending on the directional flow of water and how much of your body you have submerged in water. When it comes to building muscles, resistance can make a difference because your muscles have to counter the resistance, which in turn causes them to be stronger.

The best part is that the muscles you build will be what we call lean muscle mass, which are muscles formed after burning all excess body fat.

5: *Helps build endurance*

As discussed previously, water aerobics is a form of resistance training that challenges your muscles. The more you challenge your muscles, the stronger they get, and the bigger they become.

As your muscles become stronger and bigger, the higher your endurance becomes. Muscles are funny that way: the more you exercise them, the stronger you get, and the more you can endure the exercises.

Moreover, water aerobics is a form of light cardiovascular exercise, especially when you move quickly. The more you exercise your heart and lungs through water aerobics, the more the blood and oxygen flow to your muscles. When your muscles get more blood and oxygen, the longer you can handle strenuous activities/exercises.

Overall, the more you engage in water aerobics, the more you strengthen your muscles, and the higher your endurance becomes.

6: It is a great cardio workout

With water aerobics, the increased resistance of the water, combined with strenuous and quick movements such as running, can cause your heart to pump very fast.

When your heart pumps faster, it means you are exercising it, and like any other muscle, the more you exercise your heart, the stronger it becomes. Since your heart is responsible for some of the most important functions in your body, making it stronger will improve various other functions.

For instance, having a healthier heart will help pump oxygen and blood more efficiently, thus improving your physical performance, relieve high blood pressure, and reduce the chances of heart attacks or other cardiovascular diseases.

When it comes to high blood pressure, water aerobics can do more than relieve the condition; they can also help reduce the risk of the problem. The buoyancy of the water affects your blood flow by allowing it to flow freely and easily, thus reducing your heart rate and your blood pressure.

The same case applies to your lungs: the stronger they are, the more oxygen they can absorb and process, which means there will be a sufficient supply of blood and oxygen to your muscles, which is essential to their functionality. The healthier your lungs are, the longer you can exercise without feeling winded quickly.

7: It helps reduce stress and anxiety

Another reason why you should engage in water aerobics is that it helps reduce stress and anxiety, which means it can also help put you in a better mood.

First of all, water has shown to have a soothing effect on the mind; there is something very relaxing about the calm and serene nature of water. Evidence of this is in the fact that exercising, combined with the soothing nature of water, causes your brain to produce feel-good hormones that influence your mood.

Some of the hormones produced are endocannabinoids, a substance found in marijuana, and that is responsible for the sense of relaxation and happiness, and that helps counteract pain sensitivity. Water aerobics cause your brain to produce these hormones naturally.

Furthermore, water aerobics causes your brain to produce neurochemicals called endorphins that cause you to have a sense of relaxation, joy, and happiness. This feeling counteracts the grief and sadness caused by depression and anxiety.

That shows that the soothing nature of water can help alleviate stress and anxiety.

#: Helps keep you cool

Something great about water aerobics is that it keeps you cool and relaxed at all times, which is something we cannot say for most other forms of exercise. Staying cool is particularly important if you sweat a lot and are prone to overheating. Different forms of exercise increase your body temperature because you are pushing your body beyond what it considers its "normal" operational mode.

When you work out on dry land, especially on a hot sunny day, you are most likely going to become sticky and uncomfortable, which can cause you to feel less motivated with the workout.

Water aerobics dictates that you exercise inside the water. That means the water will cool you down as you continue working out. It will also eliminate sweating, which is usually very uncomfortable, thus motivating you to keep going.

Furthermore, the water massages and soothes your muscles in a way that leaves you feeling cool and relaxed.

These are some of the major benefits you stand to gain from engaging in water aerobics, especially as a senior. Besides these benefits, the activity is fun to indulge in, which makes it more probable that you will keep engaging in it without getting bored or giving up.

Having looked at the many benefits of water aerobics, let's discuss how to get started easily:

Section 2: Getting Started With Water Aerobics

As is the case with every other exercise-based activity, before indulging in water aerobics, you need to prepare and get ready.

In this regard, there're several vital aspects you need to keep in mind as you get started so that they can guide your way forward and motivate you to keep going.

Here now is a list of tips you need to keep in mind as you think about getting started with water aerobics:

Start small

One of the most important things you need to know before beginning water aerobics is that you need to start small. If you engage in strenuous water-based exercises right off the bat, you are going to end up feeling drained and are likelier to quit after a short.

Additionally, you should not be in a hurry to do all the exercises in one day. Remember that the resistance of the water will make moving your legs and arms more challenging than usual. If you try to exercise too much, you can easily strain your muscles.

Instead of going ham, start doing basic exercises that do not require too much effort. Doing this will help you get acquainted with the new environment and give your body time to start getting used to the exercises slowly.

Before moving to the more technical ones, start with the basic and easy exercises, and then gradually move onto advanced exercise as your body becomes stronger.

Set exercise goals

Something else you need to do before joining water aerobics is to clarify and write down your exercise goals. These exercise goals are essential because they will help you track your progress; they will also motivate you to keep taking steps forward.

Create short-term goals—what you expect to gain from engaging in water aerobics in the short-term, like a month—and long-term goals—what you expect to gain from engaging in this form of exercise in the long run. Clarifying this will help you figure out your short and long-term exercise goals.

Once you figure out the goals, write them down so that you don't forget or lose track of them. You can record them in a journal or diary.

Once you accomplish a goal, no matter how small it is, tick it off your list, which will help you see if the exercises are helping you in any way and how much you've gained from them.

Water aerobics essentials

Before you can dive into water aerobics, you will need several essential things. Without these essentials, you cannot be able to participate in the exercises.

- You can only engage in water aerobics in water that is waist-high or even deeper, which means you will need a pool that has enough water.

- Since you will need to be in the water to conduct the exercises, you will need a comfortable one-piece fitness suit/attire that covers the areas you want hidden. Such a suit will ensure you are comfortable during the workout, and that you don't have to worry about the costume coming off as you work out.

- You will also need water shoes that can help cushion the contact between your feet and the floor, failure to which can lead to blisters and irritation.

- Consider getting a waterproof cap and goggles that can help protect your hair and eyes from water damage.

- Finally, once you become a pro at water aerobics, you can consider adding water barbells, a weight belt, kickboards to help increase your weight and resistance.

These are the most important things you need to consider before engaging in water aerobics. Having them in mind will help you make a smooth transition that will make the process fun and productive.

Before every workout session, you also need to warm-up.

Here are warm-up exercises you can engage in to prepare yourself for the main water aerobics workout session:

Warm-Up Exercises For Water Aerobics

As is the case with any form of exercise, to avoid injury or complications, always warm-up before engaging in water aerobics.

Warming up is essential because of the following reasons:

- It increases blood flow to your muscles, which helps prepare them for the workout that is about to happen.

- It gradually increases your heart rate, which in turn increases blood flow, which improves your body functions in readiness for physical exertion.

- It helps prevent any injuries that may occur from sudden movements.

- It prepares you psychologically for the workout that is about to happen.

At normal water temperature, warming up should last anywhere between 5-10 minutes, depending on the intensity of the warm-up in which you are engaging.

Warm-up exercises

With your gear in place, get ready to jump into these 10-minutes workout exercises that can help you warm up before the actual water aerobics exercises:

- **Punches:**

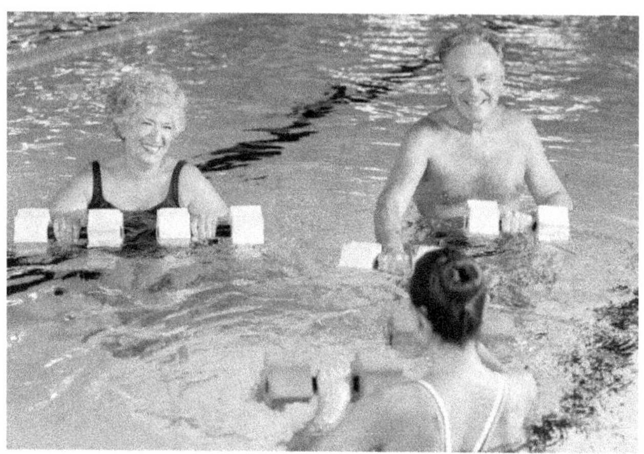

For one minute, stand with your feet shoulder-width apart and your knees slightly bent. Throw alternating punches in front of you.

- **Side steps**

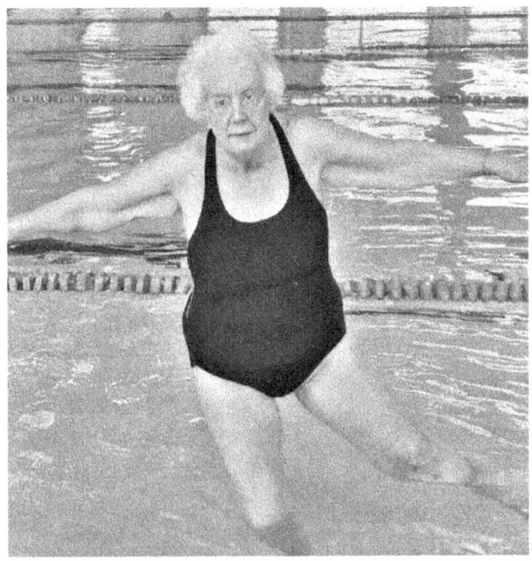

While inside the pool, move perpendicularly to your right then to your left for one minute.

- **Jumping jacks**

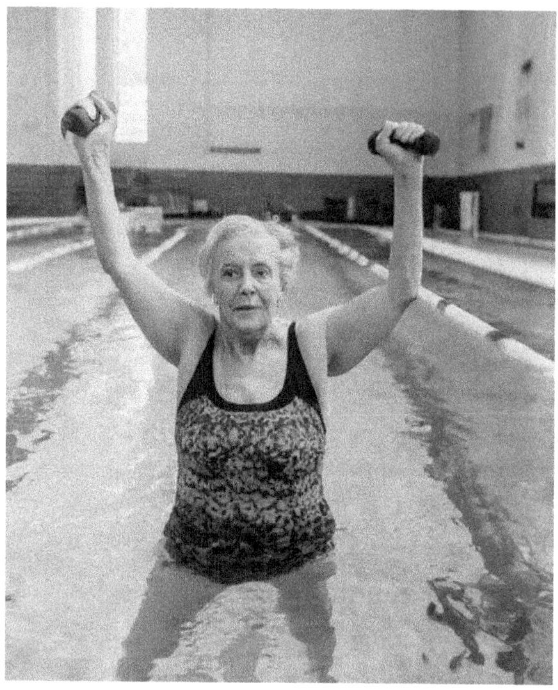

This exercise will require you to submerge yourself in the water completely, raise your arms close to the surface, then bring them back to your side. Do this for 30 seconds.

- **Tummy touch**: Begin by bringing your legs shoulder-width apart, with your knees slightly bent. With your hands out, bend your elbows at your side and keep your palms open. Maintain your elbows at your side, move your hand against the water, and then touch your stomach. Repeat the procedure with the other arm for about 1 minute.

- **Arm circles**

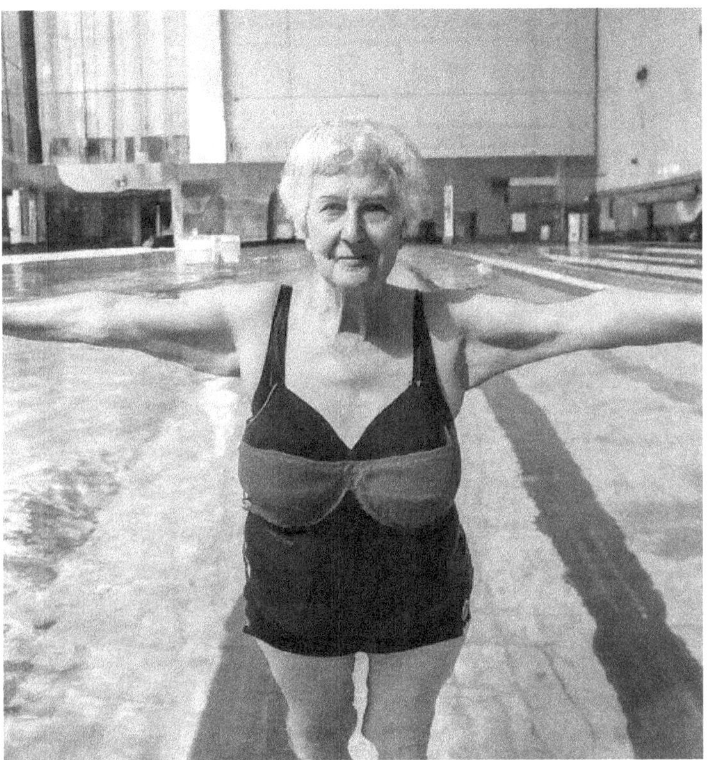

Start by jogging on the spot while making small forward circles in the water, then gradually make larger arm circles for 30 seconds.

- Jog on the spot for about 30 seconds.

- **Jump rope:**

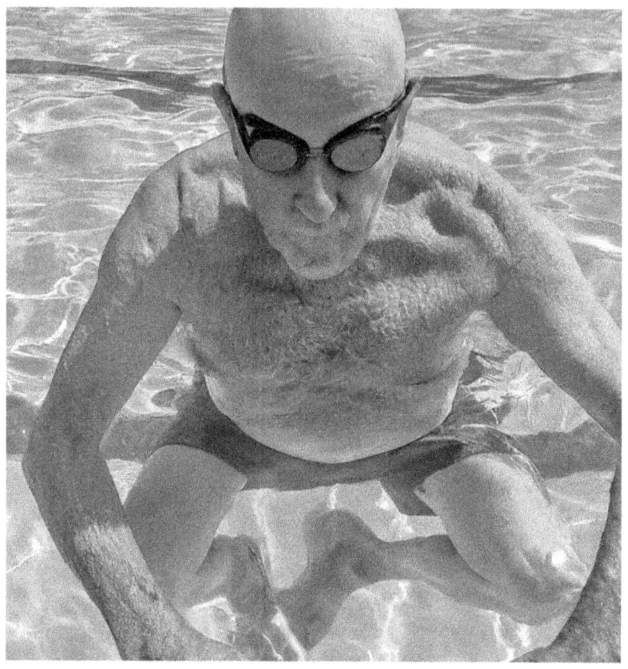

While inside the water, imagine you are jumping a rope and do that for about 30 seconds.

- **Rocking horse**

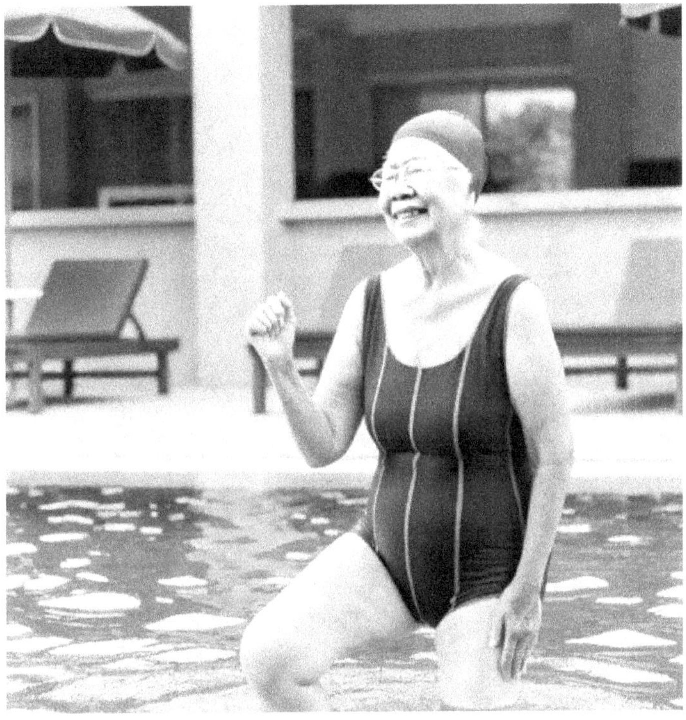

Place one foot in front of you and the other behind you, then, keeping your back foot off the ground, jump onto your front foot. Switch by keeping your front foot off the ground and jump onto your back foot. Do this for 30 seconds before switching your foot position and repeating for 30 seconds.

- **Cross country ski**

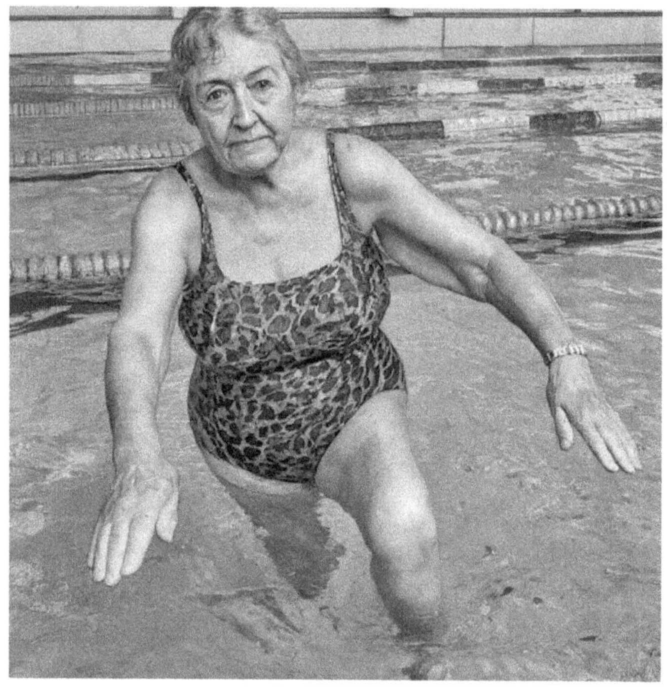

Place one arm and leg in front and the other arm and leg to the back. Assume a position that imitates cross country skiing. Keep your arms under the water and remain in that position for 30 seconds.

- **Reverse arm circles:** Jog on the spot, then using your arms, make small, backward circles with your arms inside the water before progressing to bigger arm circles for 30 seconds.

- Combine jumping jacks and cross country ski for 30 seconds each.

Rest for a short while, shake it off, then get ready to engage in the main workout. Remember to take it easy, especially if you are a senior; don't strain yourself too much: slow and sure wins the race.

Now that you have warmed up, it is time to begin your workout session:

Section 3: Water Aerobic Exercises For Seniors

The benefits of these water aerobic exercises are so many that you should feel motivated to try out most of them, if not all.

The exercises fall into two categorized sections: easy and simple, and then advanced exercises. Let's start with the first set:

Easy and Simple Exercises

The exercises in this category are easy to execute because they don't entail strenuous movements, and you don't need equipment to complete them.

1: Leg swings

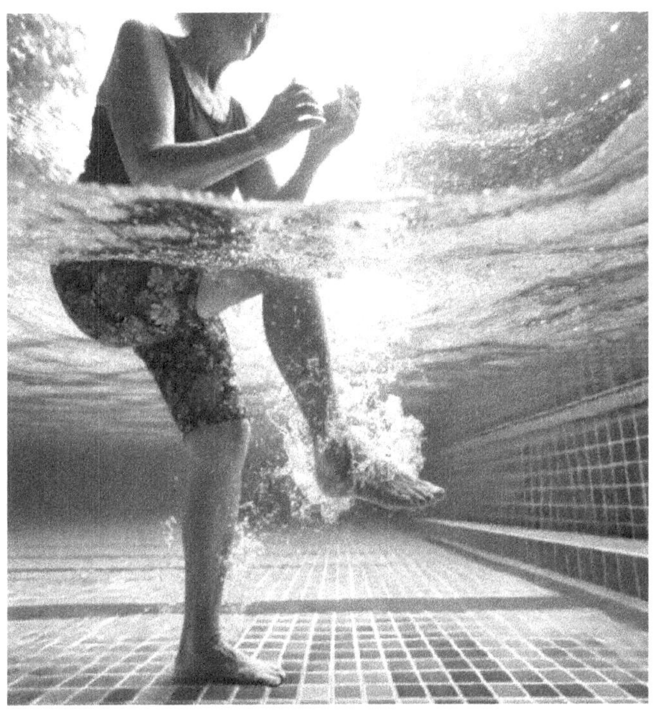

If you are looking to strengthen your leg muscles, especially your upper leg muscles, and make your hips strong and flexible, you should try out leg swings. This exercise strengthens your abdominal muscles too.

Here is how you execute the exercise:

- Begin by standing at one side of the pool while making sure that the water is deep enough to reach your lower back.

- Use your arms to hold on to the edge of the pool.

- Raise one of your legs forward and remain in that position for about 5 seconds while making sure your other leg is straight.

- Now swing the same leg sideways and hold for five seconds.

- Repeat the same procedure in both directions 12 times before doing the same process with your other leg.

2: *Flutter kicks*

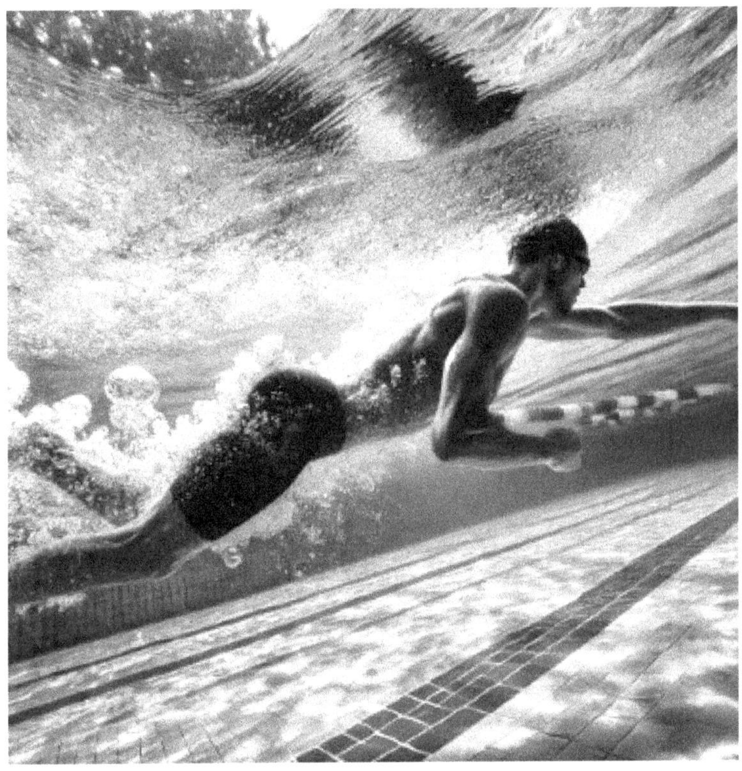

Flutter kicks are easy and very good, especially for seniors, because they are a low-impact exercise.

This exercise routine can help raise your heart, which, in turn, can help strengthen your heart. The workout is also a great way to strengthen your leg muscles and improve their flexibility. For this exercise, you can use a kickboard, but you can also do it without one. Here is how you do it:

- **If you don't use a kickboard:** Suspend your body so that you can perform a front float, keeping your head above the water, then hold on to the side of the pool. After that, make flutter kicks with your legs submerged in the water.

- **If you're using a kickboard:** Hold the kickboard in front of you, then perform a front float while keeping your head above the water. Make flutter kicks with your legs inside the water for about a minute or two.

It doesn't matter whether you use a kickboard or not; just make sure you kick at a steady pace to avoid tiring yourself out.

3: *Swimming*

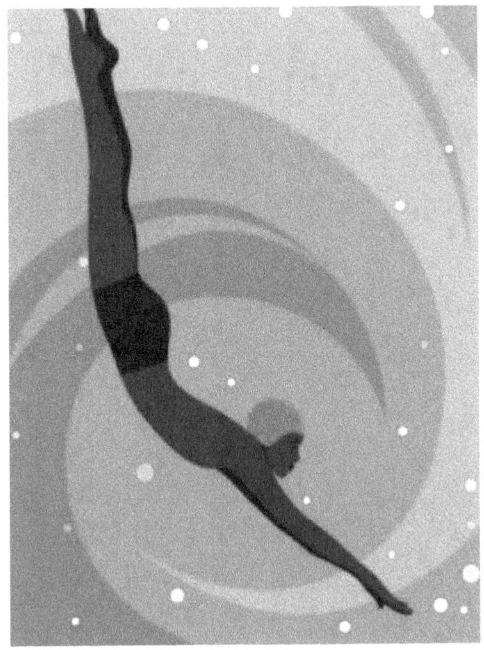

Yes, swimming is a great aerobic water exercise that many people take for granted. Swimming helps improve your muscle strength and tone and is also a great cardiovascular workout.

Swimming is a low-impact exercise that can help you lose weight because you can burn as much as 600 calories per hour. The best part is that it works out most of your muscle groups and improves your lungs and heart capacity.

Although swimming is a great workout routine that has many benefits, for it to be effective, you need to swim several laps around the pool at a steady pace. Leisurely swimming may be enjoyable, but it will not help you get the most out of the exercise.

4: Chest fly

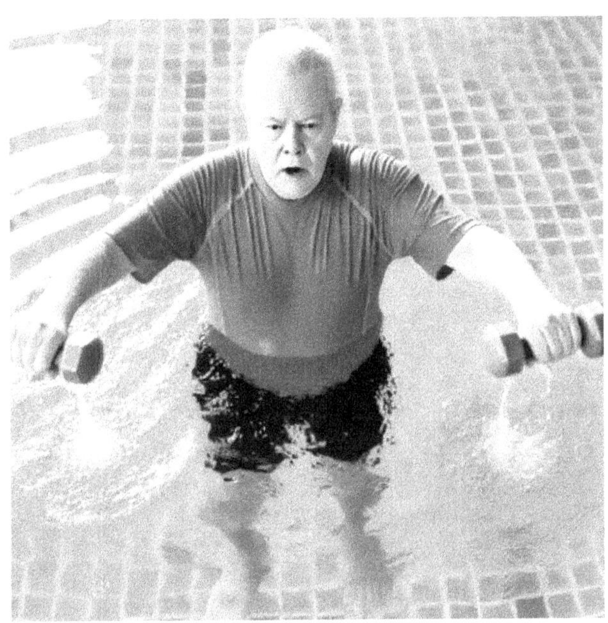

When brought to the pool, this classic gym exercise has many benefits, like minimizing the impact on your joint and bones.

You can perform chest flys with water weights or without the weights. The weights, however, will be an added advantage as it will help you maintain or build your general strength. Here is how you execute it.

- Begin by standing in a pool that has chest-high water.

- Bring your arms in front of you. Your palms should face each other and sit just below the surface of the water.

- Now push your arms towards your side then slowly push them back to the center.

- Repeat the same procedure ten times.

5: Arm curls

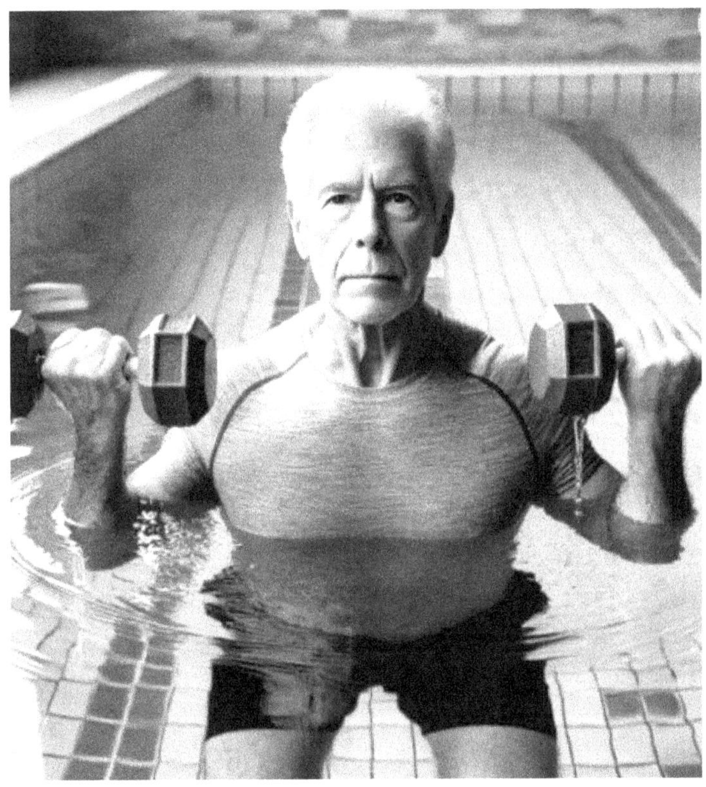

Arm curls are a great exercise that can help maintain your upper body strength. To do this workout routine, you will need a pair of water weights to increase the efficiency of the exercise.

Here is how you perform it:

- Stand in the middle of the pool with your palms facing out, holding the weights directly in front of you.

- Lift the weights in a curl and then back down. Repeat the same procedure until your arms tire out.

- You can also perform this exercise with your palms facing towards you such that it is like a conventional bicep curl exercise. The resistance offered by the water makes the exercise very effective.

6: *Water marching*

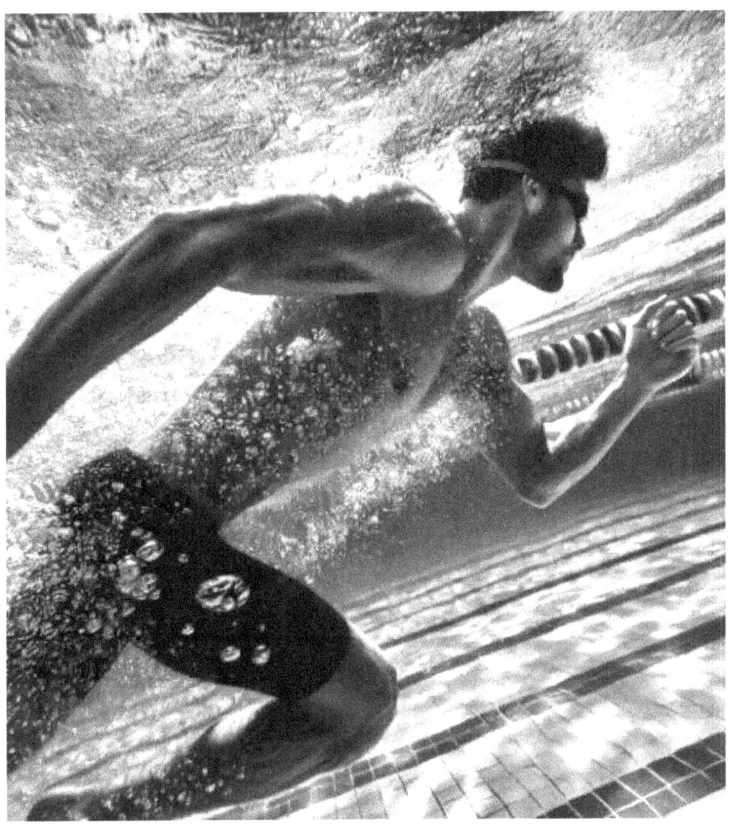

This exercise is great because it involves the whole body instead of a specific group of muscles.

Water marching helps get your heart pumping, which increases blood flow in your body. Because it's a whole-body exercise, it can improve your body functions as well as your physical appearance. The resistance provided by the water will make the exercise more effective, which will help you build up your strength.

To perform this exercise, you are going to need a spot where the water reaches your chest. Here is how to do the exercise.

- March while standing straight on the spot, and extend your legs and arms as far as you can.

- Make sure you keep your toes pointed and move your arms with energy.

- Continue marching on the spot until you feel tired.

- You should aim for a rhythmic march while keeping a steady pace.

7: *Arm circles*

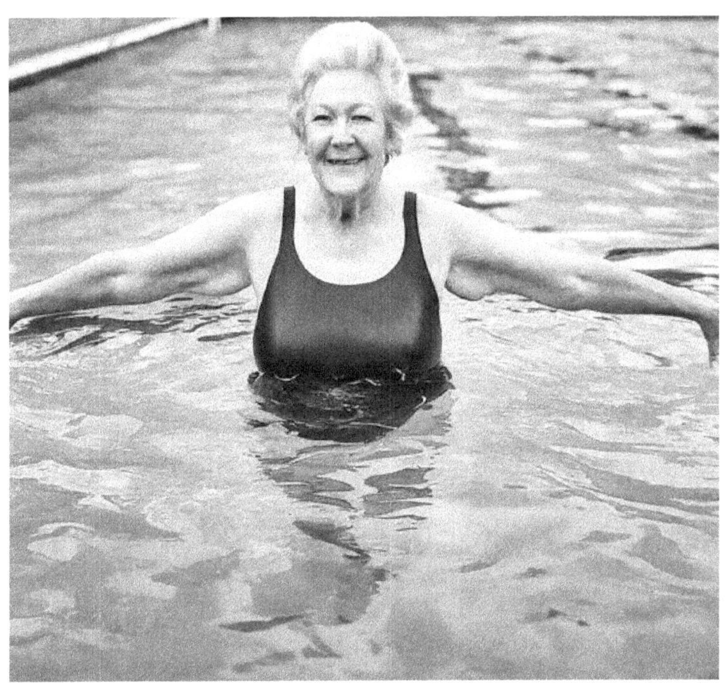

Besides being a great warm-up exercise, arm circles are also a great workout routine you should try.

The exercise can help strengthen your shoulders and upper back and your upper body muscles as a whole; it is also fun to do. Because of the energy expenditure, it can raise your heart rate, which increases blood flow to your muscles.

To do this exercise, you need to be at the edge of the pool. Make sure that you are at a depth where water goes up to your neck. You can stand at the edge of the pool to help you with balance when necessary.

Here is how you execute the exercise.

- While standing straight, put one foot in front of you and the other foot behind you.

- Lift both your arms until they are just below the surface of the water.

- Keep your palms down and your arms straight.

- Make circular motions with your arms, starting with small circles, then gradually increase the size of the circle.

- Continue making circular motions for about 10-15 seconds in one direction before repeating the same procedure in the opposite direction.

8: High-knee lift extensions

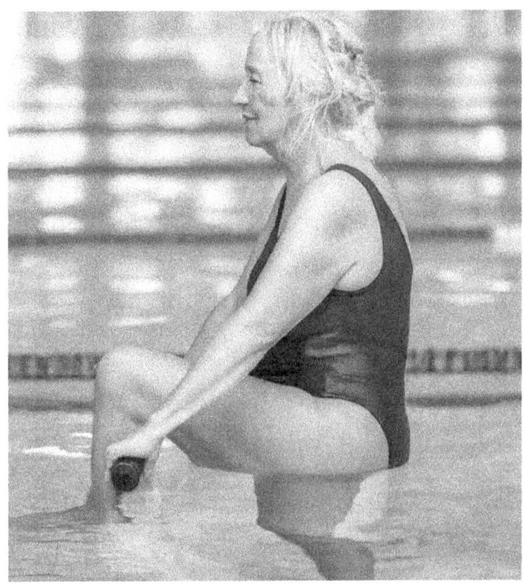

This exercise can help strengthen your lower body and core. The practice can also greatly improve your flexibility, especially in your legs. Furthermore, the exercise increases your heart rate, thus increasing blood flow to your muscles.

To perform this exercise, you need to be in chest-high water and standing at the edge of the pool in case you lose balance. If you want to make the exercise more productive, add ankle weights.

Here is how you perform the exercise.

- While standing in the pool, lift your right leg while bending your knee until your leg is at the same level as the water.

- Remain in that position for a few seconds.

- Carefully and slowly lower your leg down while keeping it straight.

- Repeat the same procedure with your left leg and continue for about 5 to 10 minutes.

9: Standing water pushups

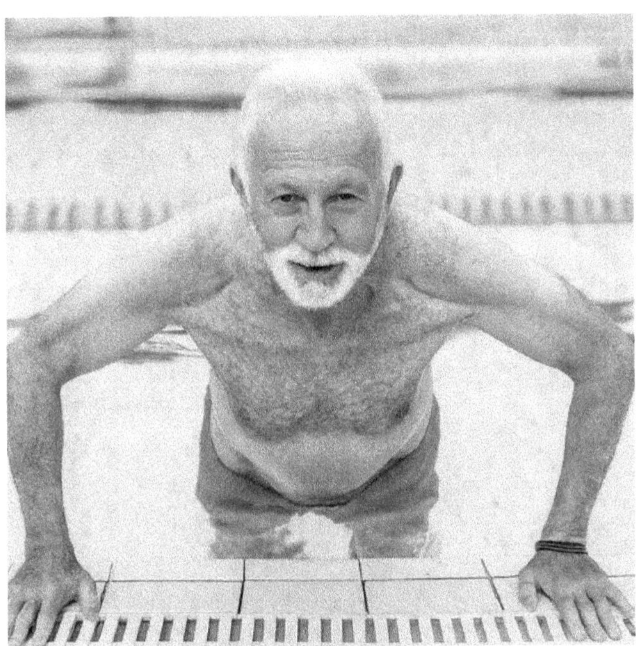

This exercise is excellent because it helps build your chest, arms, and shoulder muscles. It is quite good, especially for seniors, because it does not exert too much pressure on the joints.

Here is how to execute it:

- Stand at the edge of the pool, in chest-high water.

- Place your arms a bit wider than your shoulder width on the gutter or side of the pool.

- While standing straight, bend your arms and lean in towards the wall, then slowly push your upper body down.

- Go as low as you can, then remain in that position for 5 seconds before going back up.

- Repeat the same procedure slowly until your arms feel tired.

- Be careful not to strain your arms too much.

10: Water taxi

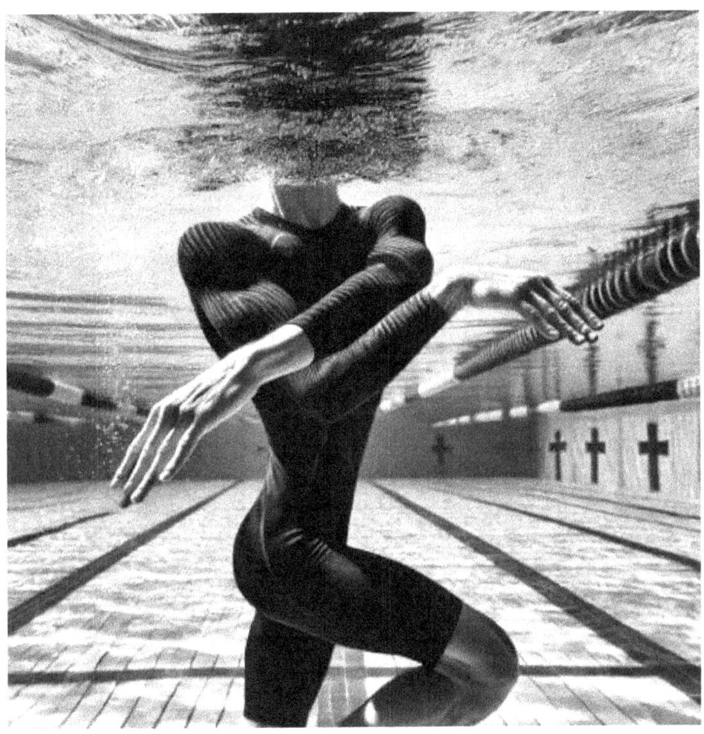

This workout routine is easy-to-do and on your joints. The exercise strengthens your shoulders, back, arms, and abs.

Here is how to execute it:

- Place your kickboard on the water and sit on it with your knees together.

- Once you sit on the kickboard, let your legs dangle inside the water.

- Bring the arms in front of you, making sure that the palms are facing away from each other. T down and diagonally outwardhen swipe your arms to your sides.

- Continue stroking your arms while in the pool for 30 seconds before switching the stroke in the opposite direction.

- Extend your arms to your sides while the palms face forward and the elbows have been bent slightly. Then proceed to sweep your arms in front of you.

- Make sure you squeeze your shoulder blades for 30 seconds throughout the exercise.

- Continue with this workout for up to 90 seconds (1 1/2 minutes) for every stroke.

11: *Tombstone kick*

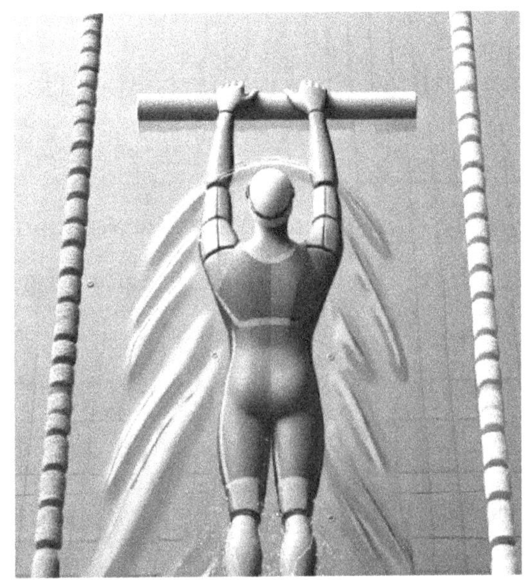

The tombstone kick is a great exercise routine that strengthens your butt, back, arms, and legs. It is also easy to do and very gentle on the joints. You are going to need a kickboard for this exercise.

Here is how to do it:

- Stand at the edge of the pool, in chest-high water.

- With your back facing the edge of the pool, place the kickboard in front of you.

- Hold it vertically using both hands such that half of it is below the surface of the water.

- Using your feet, push yourself on the surface of the water while holding the kickboard in a tombstone position.

- Kick as hard as you can with your feet inside the water for about 1 minute.

- To make the exercise more challenging and effective, hold the kickboard horizontally then completely submerge your body.

12: The Washboard

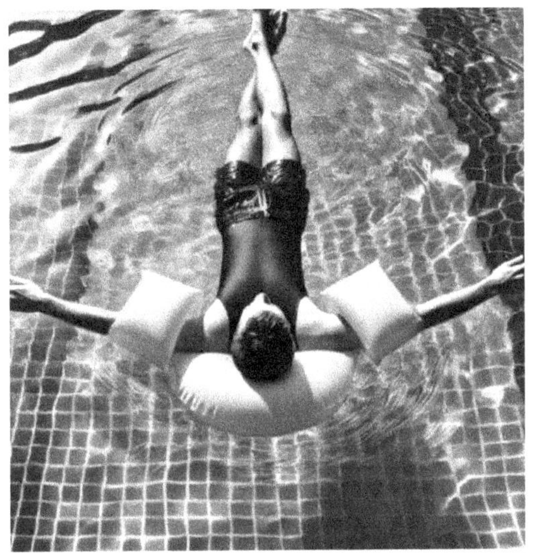

If you are looking to strengthen your arms, back, shoulders, and abs, then the washboard is the work out routine for you and is relatively easy to execute.

To execute this exercise, you will need a kickboard. Here is how to do it:

- Stand in chest-or-rib-high water, with your feet wide. Grasp both ends of the kickboard with your thumbs at the top.

- Lean forward from your hips down at an angle of 45 degrees, bend your elbows, and keep your back straight.

- Bring the board in front of your chest then push it diagonally down underwater while extending your arms and squeezing your abs.

- Use your elbows to scoop the board back like you're doing a biceps curl.

- Remain in that position for about 1 minute.

13: Deck Dip

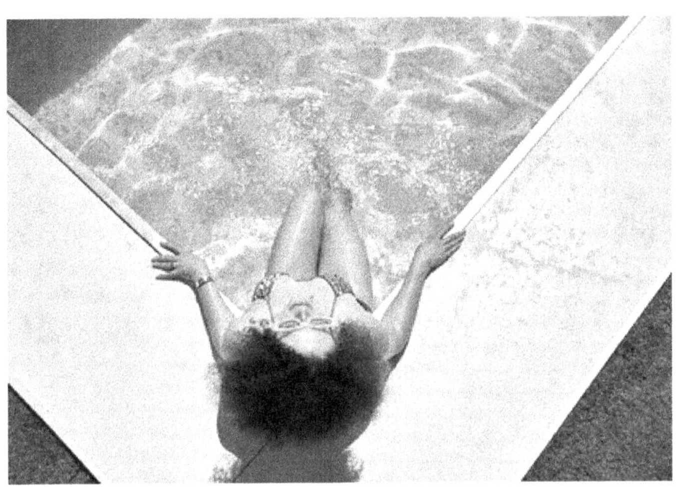

This workout routine targets your abs, triceps, and obliques. It is easy on the joints and to execute.

Here is how to perform the exercise:

- While standing in chest-high water, turn your back to the edge of the pool, and place your palms onto the edge behind you, with your fingertips facing forward.

- Now bend your left knee such that your left foot is flat against the wall.

- Next, raise your right leg until it is hip-high in front of you. Make sure it is as straight as possible.

- Straighten your arms then lift your body above the water.

- Remain in that position for about 1 minute before going down again.

- Do ten reps before changing to the right leg and repeating the same procedure.

- To make this exercise easy, keep both feet and your knees bent throughout the workout

14: *Pool edge side burpee*

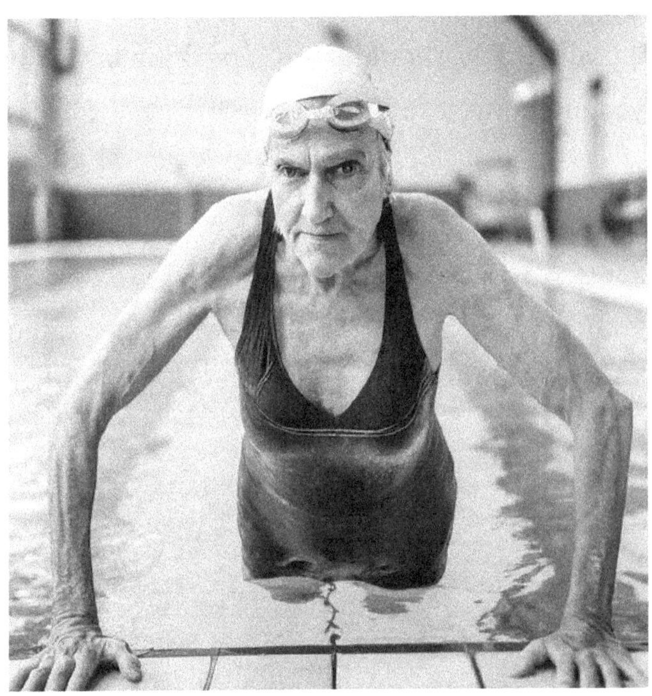

The pool edge side burpee strengthens your hips, legs, abs, and obliques. Because it's almost similar to the deck dip, this exercise is also easy to perform.

Here is how to do this workout routine:

- Once at the deep end of the pool, use your right hand to hold on to the edge of the pool; your body should be perpendicular to the wall.

- While standing straight, tuck your knees together such that your feet are flat against the wall as high as you can.

- Make sure you have a firm grip on the edge of the pool, then jump your feet off the wall and extend your legs as straight as possible. You should be in a position where it seems like you are doing a side-plank.

- Make sure you engage your abs so that they can help bring your body to the surface.

- Tuck your knees back and continue with the same procedure for one minute before switching to the other side.

15: *The Dolphin Tail*

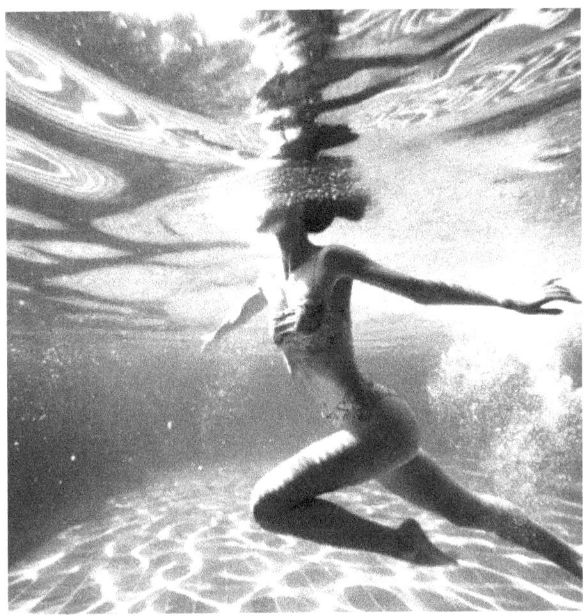

The dolphin tail is an easy workout routine that strengthens your legs and abs. It is also fun and engaging, especially for seniors, since it's easy.

Here is how to execute the exercise:

- Once in the deep end, bring your arms out to your side and extend your legs beneath you.

- Bend your knees slightly, then, while engaging your abs, squeeze your legs together and sweep them back before quickly extending them forward.

- Sweep your arms through the water to counterbalance your motion in your leg's opposite direction.

- Make sure to initiate the movement from your core, not your legs.

- Continue doing this movement for about 1 minute.

16: Vertical breaststroke

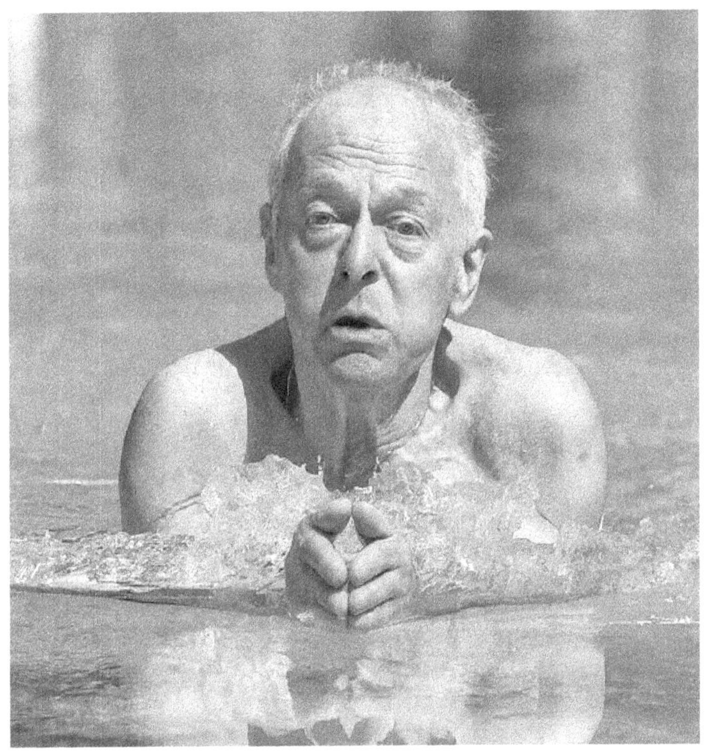

This exercise is easy on the joints and to perform too. The vertical breaststroke strengthens your hips, butt, abs, and inner thighs.

Here is how to execute it—you will need a kickboard:

- Once in the deep end, grasp both sides of the kickboard in front of you.

- Make sure to hold the kickboard above your head.

- Now extend both your legs below you.

- While flexing your feet, bend both your knees to bring your heels towards your behind.

- Next, quickly press your legs down and then diagonally outward. This should enable you to pull your body out of the water with your toes pointed.

- Finally, extend both your legs below you then repeat.

- Continue with this routine for 1 minute.

- If you find holding the kickboard above your head too difficult, you can let your arms float by your side or raise them above your head.

17: **One-legged balance**

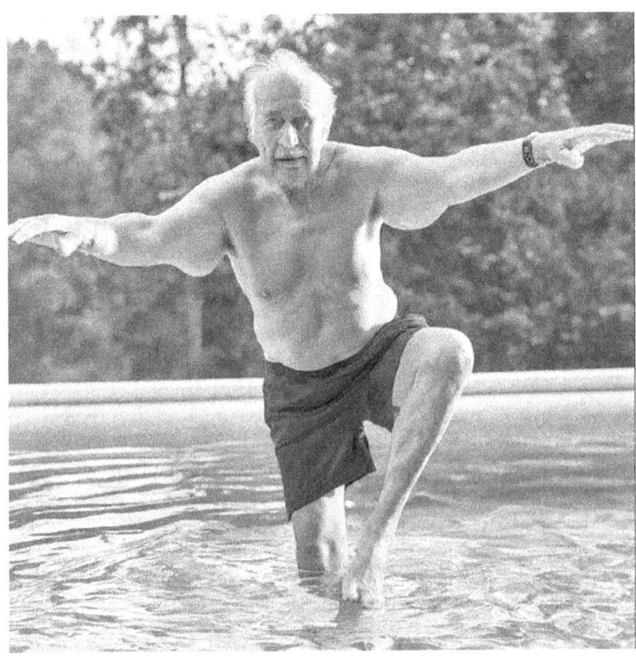

This one-legged balance exercise is perfect if you are looking to strengthen your core and leg muscles. It is a no-impact exercise, which makes it great for seniors because it removes the risk of falling or injuries.

Here is how to do it—you will need a noodle:

- Stand where the water rises up to waist high.

- Next, lift the left knee and put a noodle under the left foot (make sure you position the middle of the noodle)

- Balance your left foot on the noodle while keeping your hands by your side.

- Now move your left knee out sideways then balance for about a minute.

- Switch to the other leg and repeat the procedure while the right knee is lifted and the right foot is placed on the noodle.

- To make the exercise more challenging, place both your arms on your head as you balance. If you are with someone else in the pool, you can tell them to jog in circles to create currents that will challenge your balance.

18: Spiderman

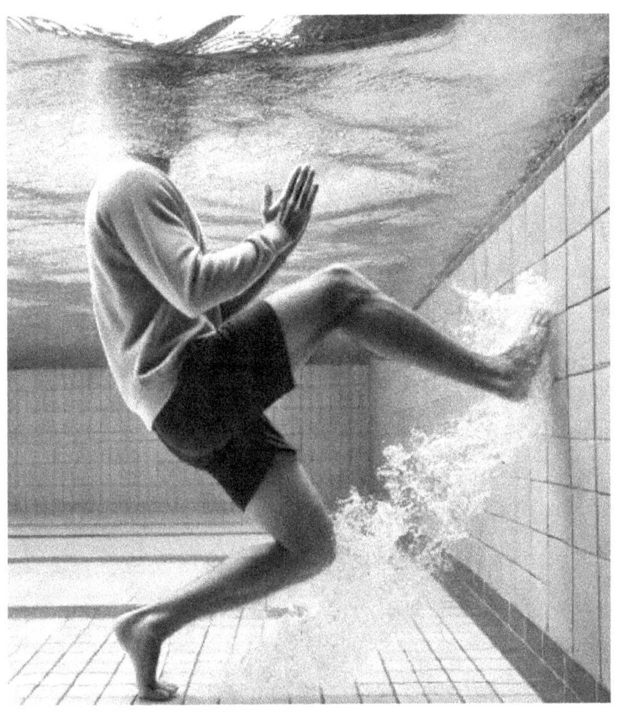

If you are a fan of Spiderman, the superhero from Marvel and DC comics, you will find this exercise fun and engaging. It allows you to climb the pool the same way Spiderman climbs buildings.

The exercise is easy and good for seniors because it defies gravity in ways not possible on land. It also strengthens the back and core muscles.

Here is how to perform this exercise:

- Start by standing at the side of the pool, in chest-high water.

- As you move your legs from the pool floor and up the side of the pool, stabilize your body by moving your arms back and forth.

- Move up and down the side of the pool and the floor as high as you can, then go back to your original position.

- Repeat the same procedure four times and alternate the lead leg each time you reach the end of one jogging circuit.

19: Chaos Cardio

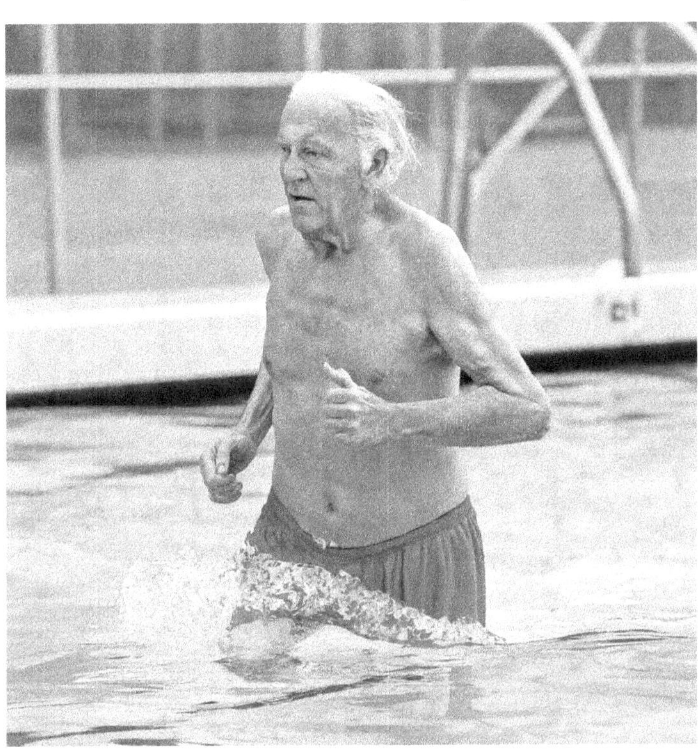

This workout routine takes jogging to a whole new level. When you create currents in the water by running through it, you strengthen your core muscles since you'll be struggling to stabilize them.

The exercise is also easy for anyone to perform. Make sure you align your ears, shoulders, and hips in one vertical line so that you can have proper alignment. That will allow you to exercise your core, not your legs or shoulders.

Here is how to do it:

- Begin by standing in waist-high water.

- Run from one end of the pool to the other end in a zigzag pattern, then immediately run straight through the currents you've created.

- Repeat the same procedure in 3-minute intervals as you alternate with something less-cardio intensive like the one-legged balance exercise.

20: Pool plank

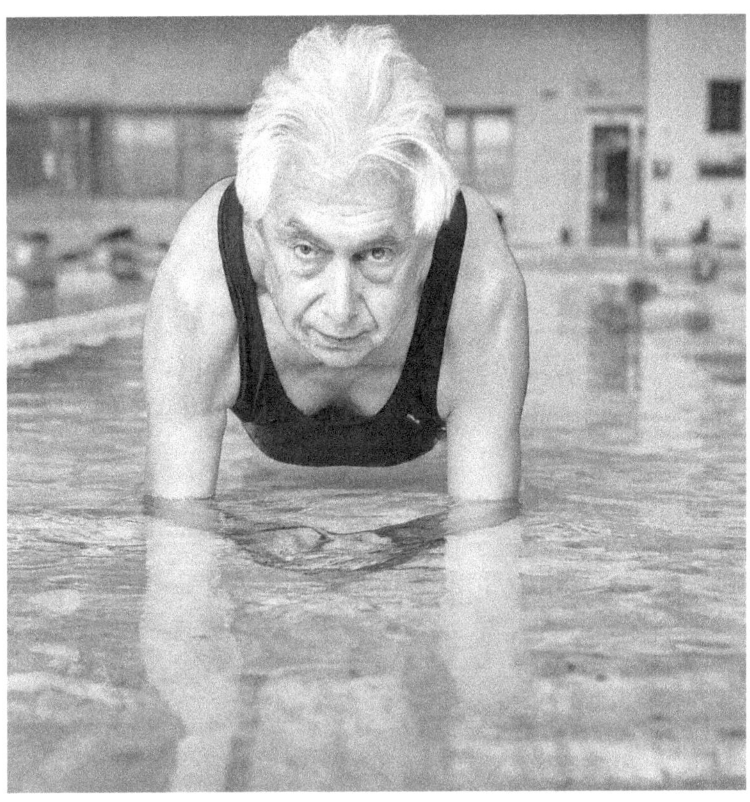

The plank is a famous exercise used to strengthen your core muscles, biceps, and leg muscles.

Planks are not easy to perform on land, especially for those who don't have strong upper muscles. All that changes in the pool because the water offers a lot of support, which is ideal because planks strengthen your core and boost your endurance.

Here is how you execute this exercise—you will need a noodle:

- Begin by standing in chest-high water.

- Use both hands to hold a noodle in front of you, ensuring the noodle is vertical.

- Press the noodle downwards into the water and then proceed to lean forward. You want to ensure your body inclines evenly.

- Try to remain stable for about 1-2 minutes.

- Repeat the procedure four times.

21: Cardio/resistance combo

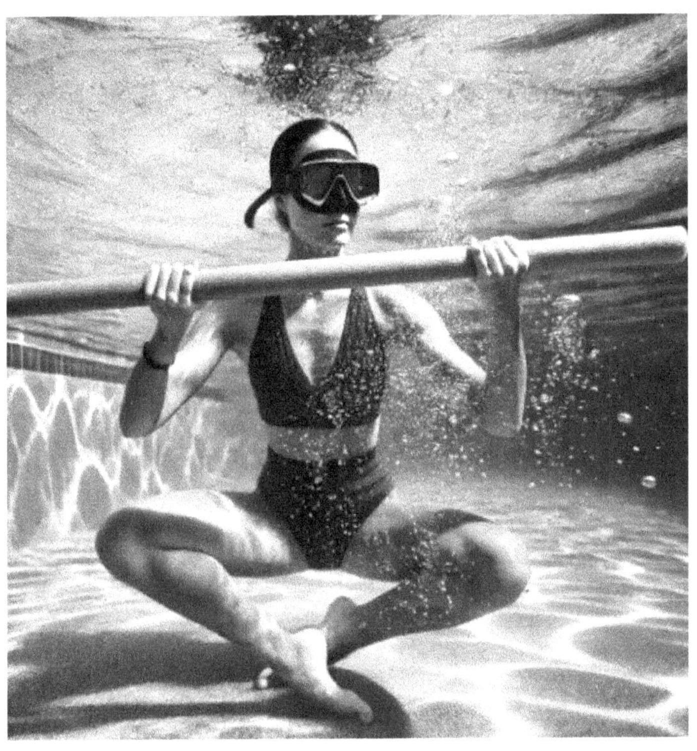

This exercise strengthens your core, upper chest, arms, and back. It also increases your heart rate, which helps burn calories. It is also easy to perform as it does not have a lot of strenuous movements. You are going to require a noodle for this exercise.

Here is how you execute it:

- Begin by standing in chest-high water.

- Place the noodle between your legs and straddle it as if you're sitting on a horse.

- Now pedal as fast as you can, making sure you open and close your arms.

- Make sure to sit upright as you perform the exercise, do not lean—this will force your core muscles to keep you stable.

- Continue with this exercise for 3 minutes.

22: *Fly backs*

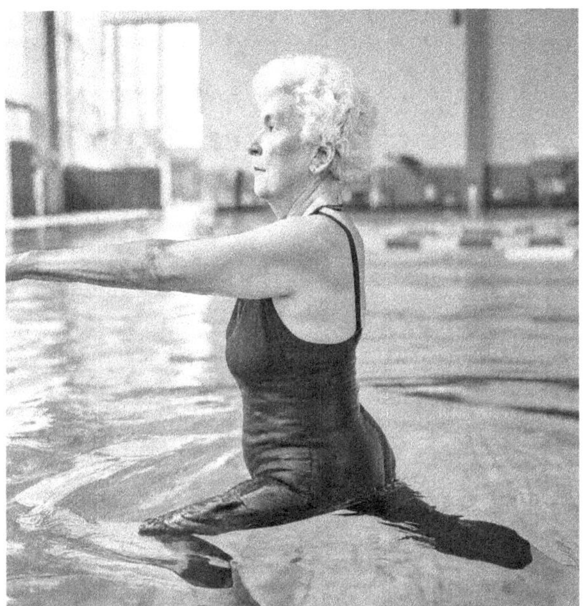

Fly backs strengthen your upper chest, arms, and back. The exercise can also improve your posture and is easy to do, which makes it perfect for all ages, even seniors.

Here is how to execute this exercise:

- Begin by standing at the center of the pool, in waist-high water.

- Get into the lunge position, ensuring the knees are bent and the left leg extends straight behind the pool.

- Now extend the arms straight out in front of you. You want to ensure the arms get to a chest height level. Make sure your palms are touching, thumbs up, and your fingers extended straight.

- Next, open your arms straight out to the sides inside the water then bring them back to their original position.

- Repeat the same procedure in four sets of 8 to 15 reps while switching the forward leg for each set.

- To make the exercise more effective or more challenging, do these reps while jogging or walking across the pool.

23: Cardio core ball running

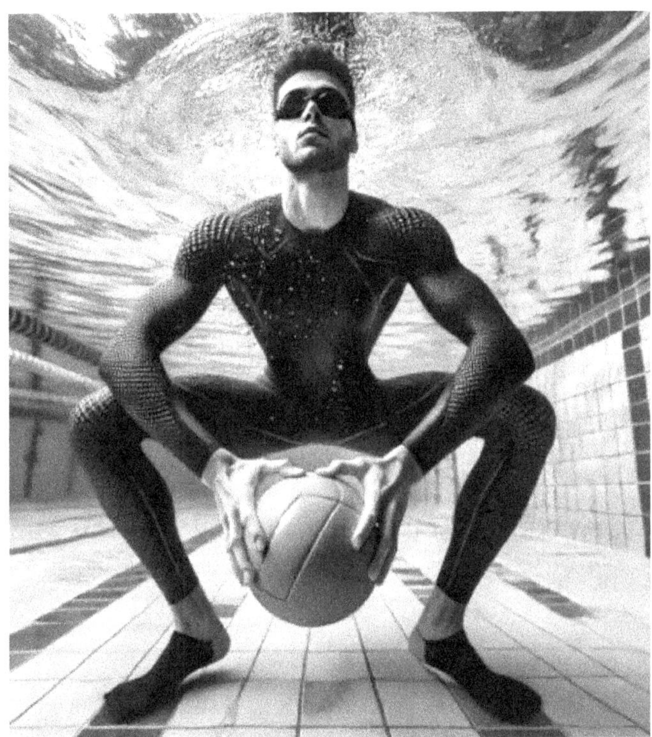

This cardio workout strengthens core muscles.

The exercise requires you to have a ball with which to add extra resistance. This ball pulls you off-center so that your core muscles have to engage so that you can keep moving forward.

You can also make the exercise more challenging by shifting the ball's position.

Here is how to execute two versions of the exercise:

Version A

- While standing in chest-high water, tuck the ball under your right arm at waist height.

- Keep your shoulders forward, and then run across the pool as fast as possible for one minute.

- Now change the ball to your left arm then run for another minute.

- Repeat the procedure four times, making sure to run faster each time.

Version B

- While standing in waist-high water, place the ball in front of your navel and hold it with both hands.

- Now run across the pool as fast as you can for about one minute.

- Rest for 30 seconds, then repeat the procedure three times, making sure to increase your speed with each rep.

24: Core ball static challenge

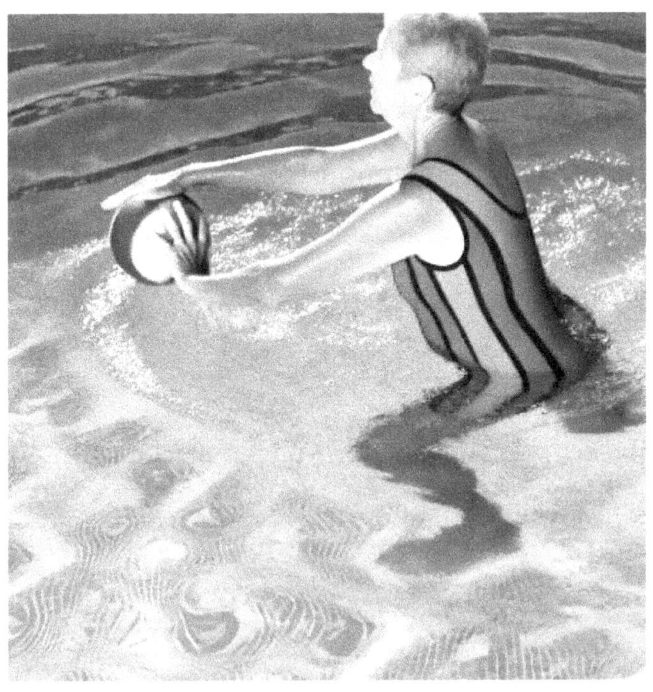

The core ball static challenge is a deceptively simple challenge that can help strengthen your core as you try to remain upright. Once you change the position of your legs and arms, it becomes four exercises in one. This exercise consists of four versions that work to achieve the same goal strengthening your core.

Here is how to perform the four versions of this exercise—you will need a ball:

Version A

- Lift your left knee as you stand in waist-high water then balance on the right knee.

- Place the ball in front of your navel, and then hold it down using both your arms for 30 seconds.

- Now repeat the procedure with your right knee lifted while standing on your left leg.

Version B

- Begin by standing in waist-high water, then assume the lunge position with your left leg extended behind you and your right leg bent.

- Now place the inflated ball in front of your navel and hold it down with both your hands directly.

- Make sure your shoulders are back and down.

- Engage your core to keep yourself upright, then remain in that position for 30 seconds.

  - Change legs then hold that position for another 30 seconds.

Version C

- While standing inside waist-high water, lift your left knee, and then balance on your right leg.

- Hold the ball in front of your navel using both arms for 30 seconds.

- Now repeat the same procedure with your right knee lifted and standing on your left leg.

Version D

- Start by standing in waist-high water, repeat the procedure detailed in version A, but this time, hold the ball with your arms outstretched.

- To have an added advantage, press the ball under the surface of the water as you workout.

25: Pushups

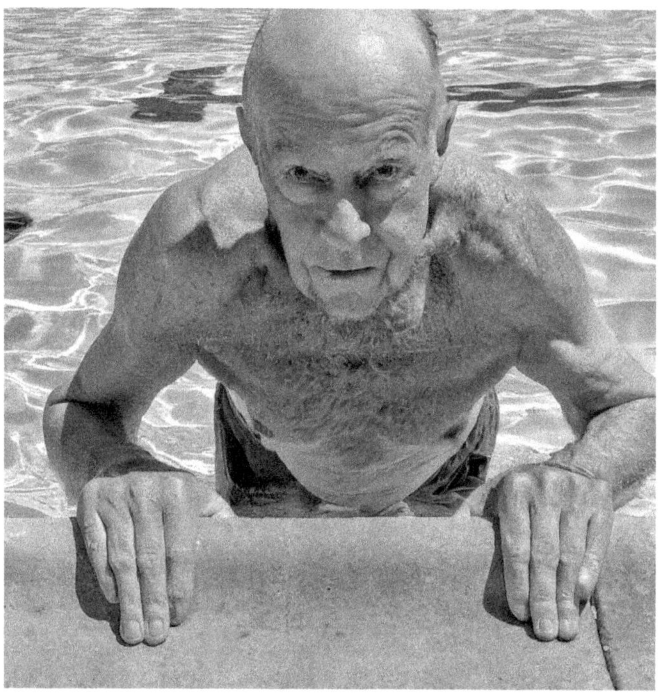

Pushups strengthen your chest, triceps, shoulders, and core.

However, this version of the pushup is different from the standard version you do on land in that you have to perform it vertically instead of horizontally. That's it's a lot easier, but the resistance from the water makes it more effective.

Here is how you can execute the exercise:

- Start by standing by the edge of the pool, in chest-high water.

- Extend your arms straight and place them on the deck at the edge of the pool.

- Make sure you are standing straight.

- Slowly lower your body towards the edge of the pool by bending your elbows to an angle of 90 degrees as low as possible, keeping your feet together.

- Once you go as low as possible, slowly go back to your original position.

- Repeat this procedure about 10-12 times until you feel the effects in your arms and core.

26: Triceps Dip

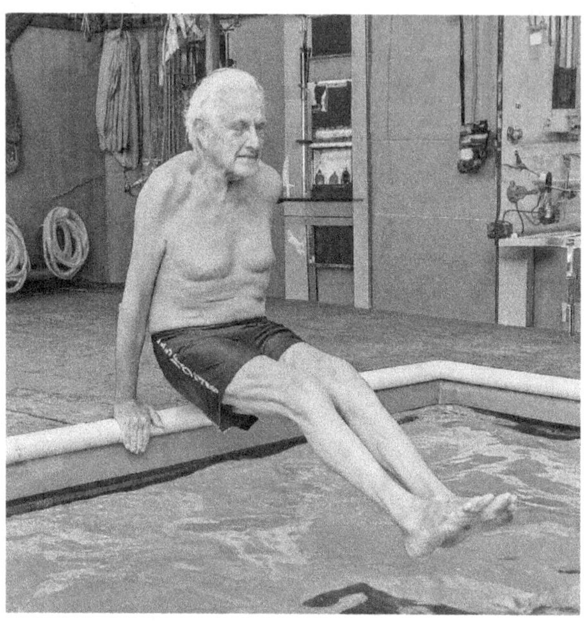

If you are looking to build your triceps and core muscles easily and fast, then the triceps dip is a great workout routine. The exercise is also easy and fun to do, making it great for everyone, but especially seniors.

Here is how to execute this exercise:

- Begin by sitting at the edge of the pool with your feet inside the water. If your feet touch the bottom of the pool, bend them and place your soles flat on the side of the pool.

- Make sure your hands grip the ledge, shoulder-width apart.

- Push your body forward, then slowly lower your body into the water until your arms form 90 degrees angle.

- Go as low as you can then slowly pull yourself up from the water to your original positions.

- Repeat the procedure for 10-15 reps.

27: Bicycle kicks

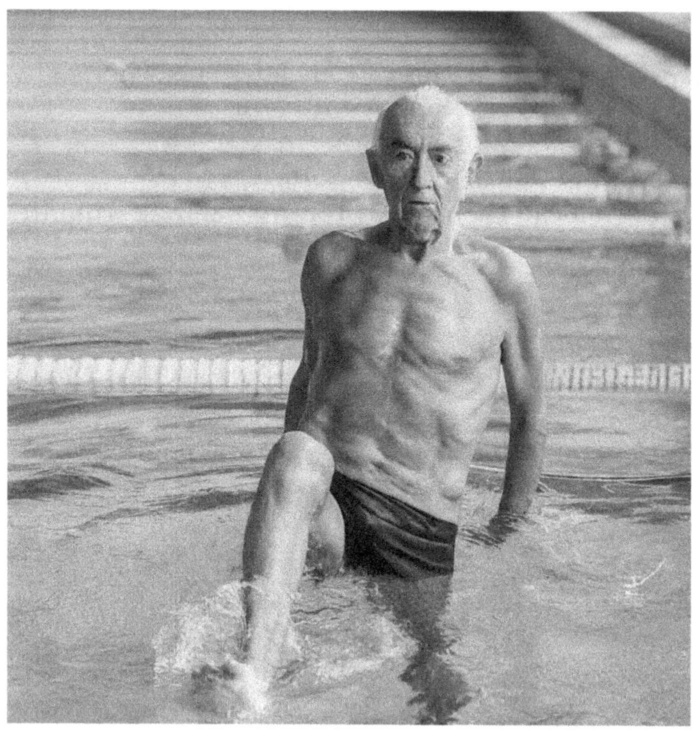

Bicycle kicks strengthen your legs, core, obliques, back, and latissimus dorsi muscles (Lats). This exercise is a bit challenging than others, but anyone who is not averse to putting in some work can do it.

Here is how you execute this exercise:

- Start by standing at the side of the pool, in chest-high water.

- Make sure that you stand with your back facing the side of the pool and your forearms on the pool ledge.

- Put your legs together, then lift them straight until hip level to an angle of 90 degrees.

- Once you assume that position, engage your abs, then bend your right knee in towards your chest and then re-extend it again before doing the same with the left leg.

- Continue alternating your legs successfully until you mimic a person peddling a bicycle.

- Repeat this procedure for about 60 seconds before resting and repeating.

28: Tuck jumps

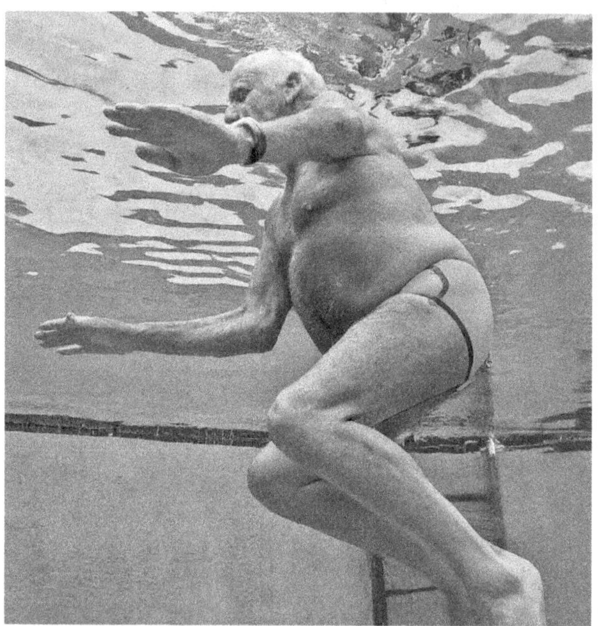

This kind of exercise is perfect for a whole-body workout and building your cardiovascular strength. Therefore, compared to steady-state cardio, you are likelier to experience an increased calorie burn. The exercise is good for people of all ages, even seniors.

Here is how to execute this exercise:

- Begin by standing in chest-high water.

- Place your feet hip-width apart, with your arms at your side.

- Now extend your arms forward at shoulder height, then bend your knees slightly.

- Make sure that you bend and widen your elbows, and that your palms are facing the water.

- Next, bend your knees and slowly lower your upper body into the water.

- Jump straight up while lifting your knees to touch your hands.

- Then land softly back in your original position with your knees bent.

- Repeat the procedure 5 to 10 times.

29: Squat jump

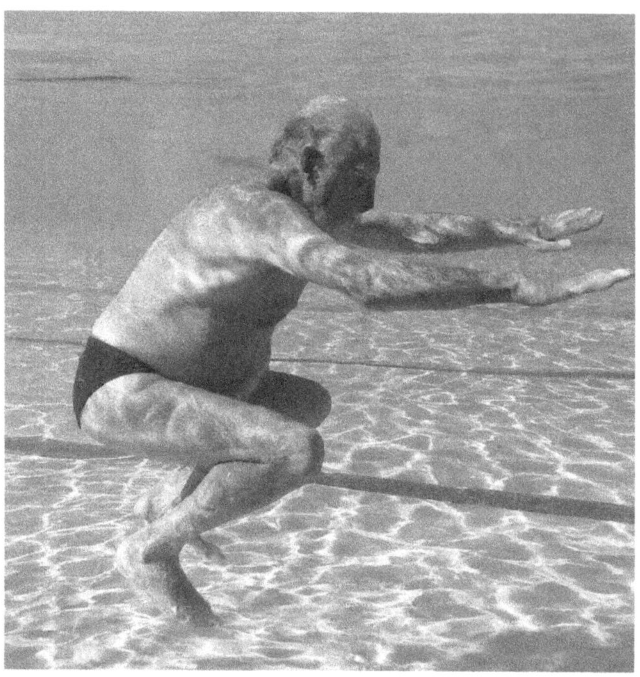

This variation of the tuck jump strengthens your upper back, shoulders, glutes, quads, and cardiovascular muscles. The squat jump is excellent because the explosive action creates a high intensity, plyometric movement, minus the impact on your joints, as is the case when performing the exercise on land. If you are looking to increase your heart rate and get in an additional upper body workout, you should involve your hands.

Here is how you execute this exercise:

- Begin by standing in waist-high water.

- Assume a low squat then extend your arms straight forward at shoulder height.

- Suddenly and explosively jump off the pool floor while pressing your arms down.

- Go back to your original position then repeat the same procedure for 12-15 times.

30: Scissor kicks

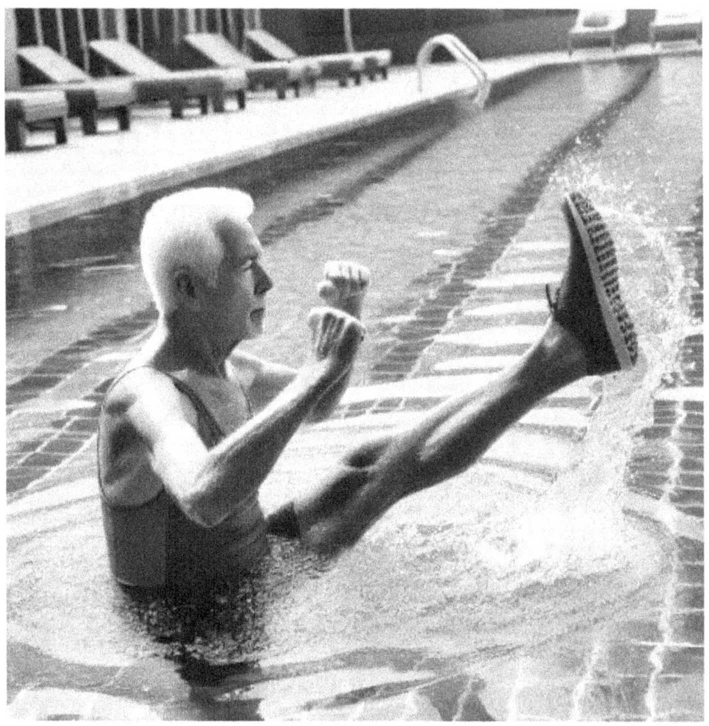

The scissor kicks exercise helps strengthens your glutes, core, inner and outer thighs. It is also easy to perform, making it suitable for all ages, even seniors. This exercise usually targets the lower body, more precisely the stabilizer muscles.

Here is how you execute this exercise:

- Begin by standing in chest-high water.

- Suspend yourself in the water and float on your stomach while using your arms to hold onto the pool's ledge.

- Extend your legs straight to form one long line.

- Make sure to engage your abs so that you can keep your torso facing downward and your hips level.

- Cross your right leg over your left leg, creating an "X" shape with your lower body.

- Go back to your original position, then repeat the same procedure with your opposite leg first.

- Continue alternating your sides for 60 seconds per set.

31: Reverse Fly

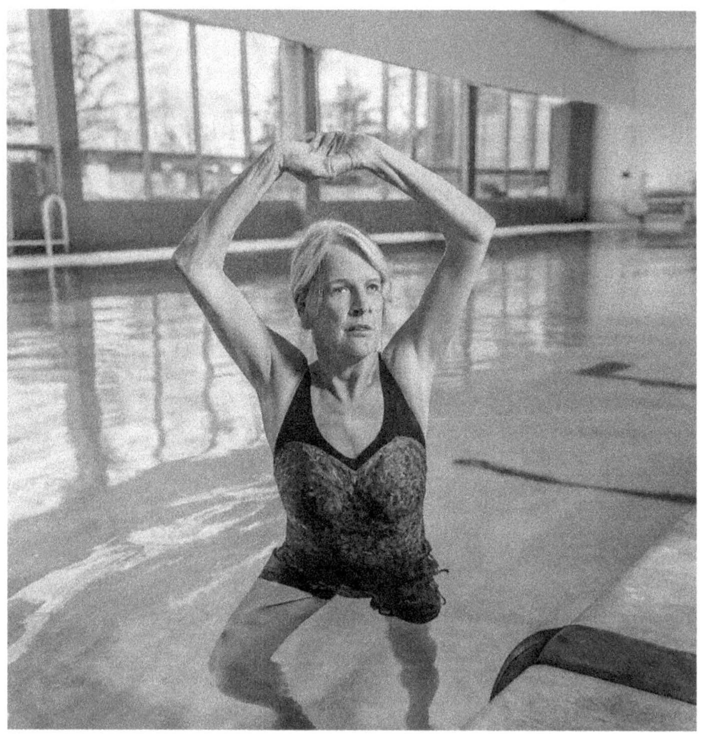

The arm workout that is part of this workout routine strengthens your quads, upper back, core, and glutes. The exercise is also easy for anyone to do because it does not entail strenuous or difficult movements.

Here is how you execute this exercise:

- While standing in chest-high water, spread your legs hip-width apart, and keep your knees slightly bent.

- Tilt your torso forward, with your arms hanging straight by your sides and your palms facing your body.

- Now raise both your arms out to your side until they reach shoulder height, then squeeze your shoulder blades together.

- Go back to your original position and repeat the procedure to complete a rep.

- Do 12-15 per side each set.

32: Plie jump squats with heel touch

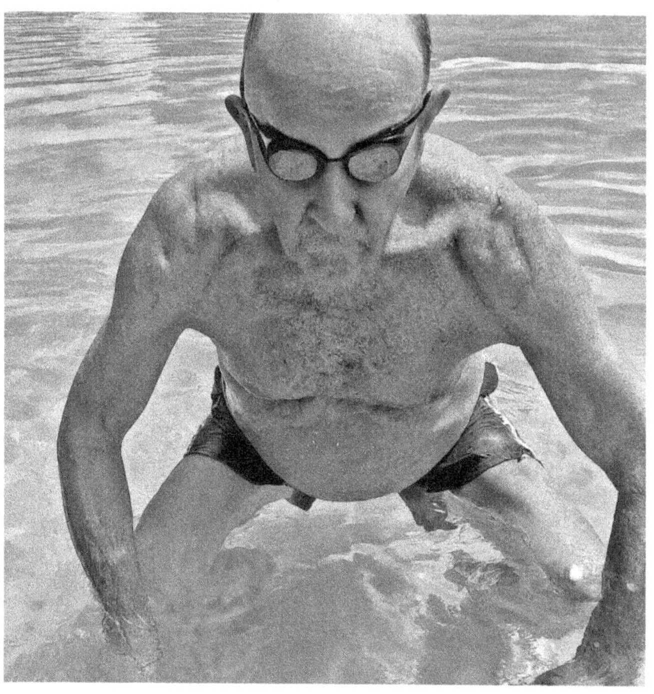

This exercise works your glutes, outer/inner thighs, and enhances your cardiovascular strength minus the impact you'd experience on solid land. Because it's a variation of the squat jumps, it's ideal for all ages, but especially for seniors who require no impact but quite practical exercises.

Here is how to do this exercise:

- Start by standing in chest-high water.

- Now spread your legs shoulder-width apart, with your toes turned out, and your arms by your side.

- Next, bend your knees, then slowly lower your upper body to assume a squat position.

- Bring your hands together straight in front of your chest.

- Quickly jump up by bringing your feet together, extend your legs straight, then bring your heels to a touching position.

- Pull your feet apart again, then land in a wide-legged squat once again.

- Continue the procedure and do 12-15 per set.

33: Lunging Torso twist

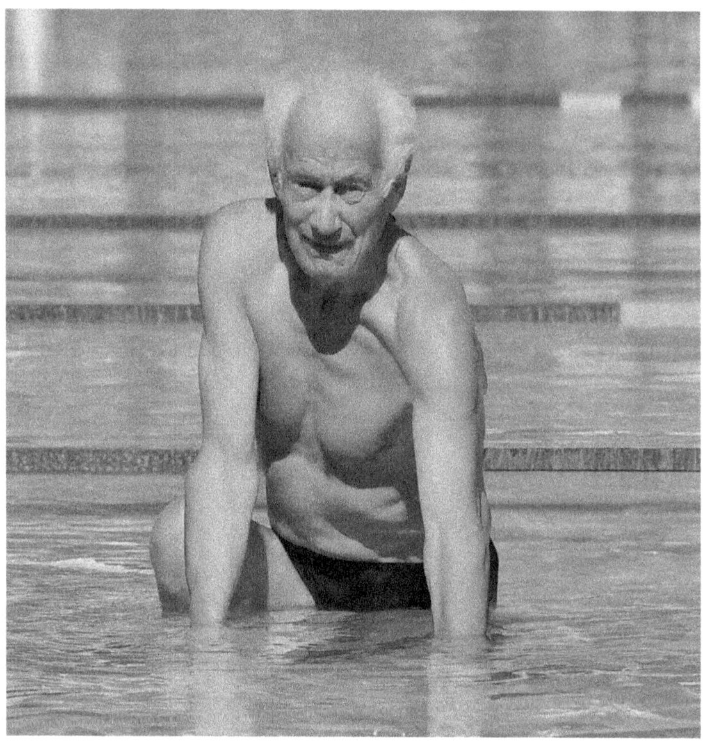

This exercise strengthens your inner thighs, obliques, glutes, and quads. It offers a staggered stance in your leg that challenges your stability while the torso rotation engages your core. The exercise is also easy to perform, making it great for seniors and people of all ages.

Here is how you execute it:

- While standing in waist-high water, place your arms at your side.

- Spread your legs apart and take a big step forward with your right leg, then lower down into a lunge.

- Make sure that you keep your head above the water and your heel as high as you can.

- Extend your arms straight at shoulder level, then twist your upper body towards the right side.

- Now go back to your original position and repeat on the opposite side, bring your left leg forward then rotate towards the left side.

- Repeat the same procedure and do 12-15 per side each set.

34: Water arm lifts

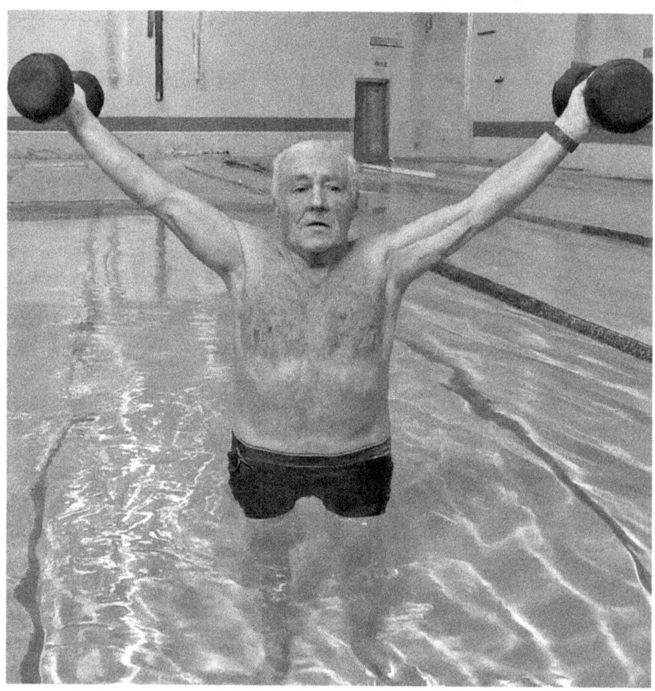

This exercise strengthens your arm muscles. It also helps to increase blood flow to your muscles, thus boosting your strength. Water arm lifts are incredibly easy for anyone—irrespective of age—to do. You will also require dumbells to add more resistance to the workout.

Here is how you perform this exercise:

- Begin by standing in shoulder-high water.

- Now pick up the dumbbells in each arm, then hold them by your side, with your palms facing upwards.

- Now bring your elbows closer to your torso as you lift your forearms until they reach the level of the water.

- Next, slowly rotate your wrists downwards.

- Gradually lower your arms back to their original position.

- Repeat the same procedure for 1-3 sets of 10-15 reps for each exercise.

35: Back Wall glide

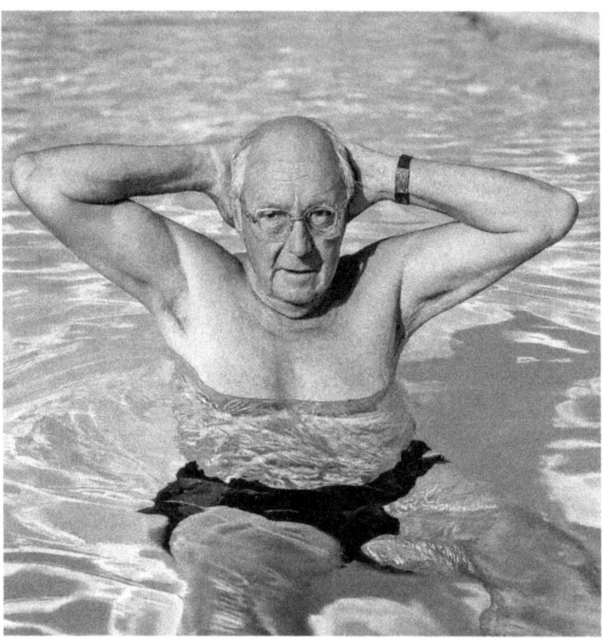

The back wall glide strengthens your core and lower body. It is also friendly on the joints and easy-to-do, which makes it suitable for all ages.

Here is how you execute it:

- Start by standing in chest-high water.

- Get a hold on the pool ledge then tuck your knees into your chest before pressing your feet into the wall.

- Now push yourself away from the wall and float gently on your back as far as possible.

- Draw your knees back into your chest, then press your feet down to the bottom of the pool, and then run back up to the wall.

- Repeat the same procedure for about 5 to 10 minutes.

36: Lateral arm lifts

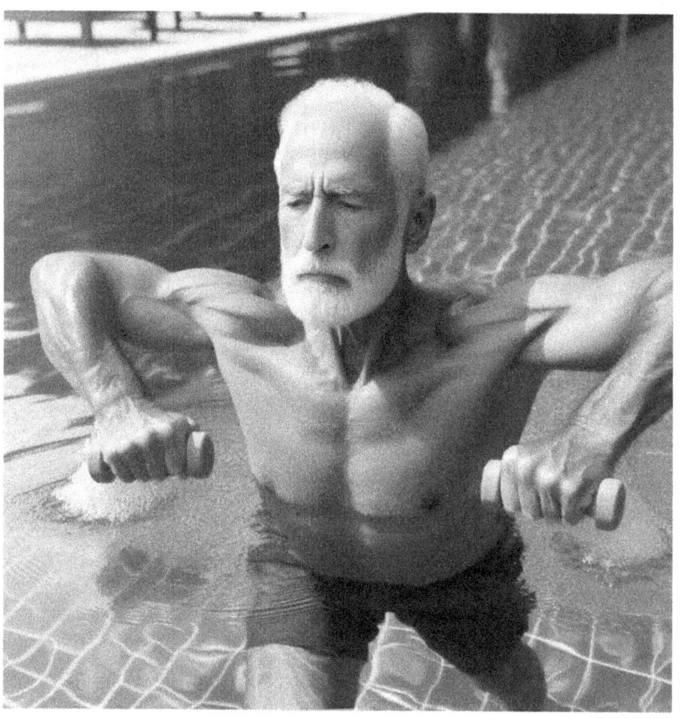

If you're looking to strengthen your upper body as a whole, then lateral arm lifts are perfect. They work out your upper body and are easy to execute, making them suitable for all ages.

You are going to require dumbbells for this exercise so that you can increase your resistance.

Here is how you execute this exercise.

- Begin by standing in shoulder-high water.

- Now take your dumbbells and hold them at your side

- Raise both arms up until they reach the same level as your shoulders and the water.

- Slowly lower your arms back down to your sides.

- Repeat the same procedure for 8-14 times.

37: Leg lifts

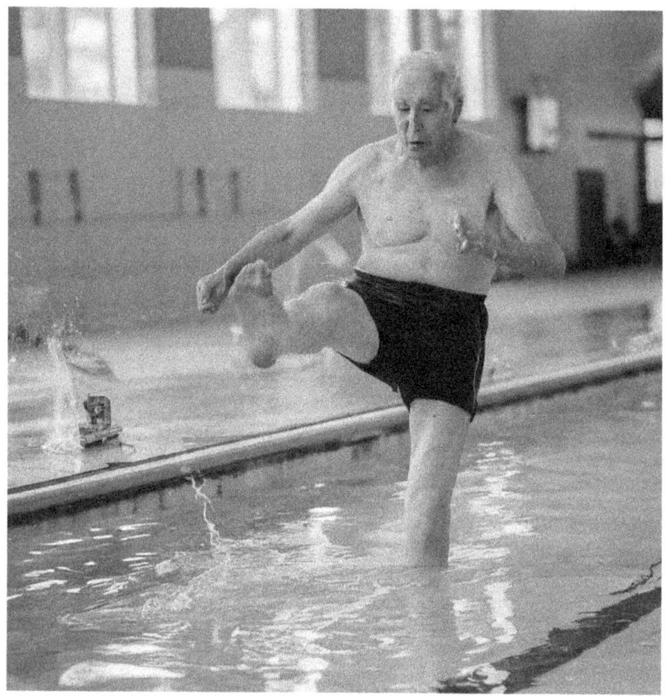

Leg lifts are a great exercise to try because besides being easy to do, they also help strengthen your core and leg muscles. The exercise requires you to remain suspended between two noodles that help you with your balance as you lift both your legs, which means that for this exercise, you are going to need two noodles.

Here is how to execute this exercise:

- Start by standing in shoulder-high water.

- Take the two noodles and place one under each arm so that you can be able to keep your head above the water.

- Once you've gained your stability, bring your legs together and lift them at once.

- Bring them as high as you can until you form a 90-degrees angle, then bring them down slowly to your original position.

- Make sure your feet don't touch the floor of the pool between each rep.

- Repeat this procedure for one minute, without rushing: slowly lift and bring your legs back.

- Continue with these movements for about ten sets.

38: Pendulum leg swings

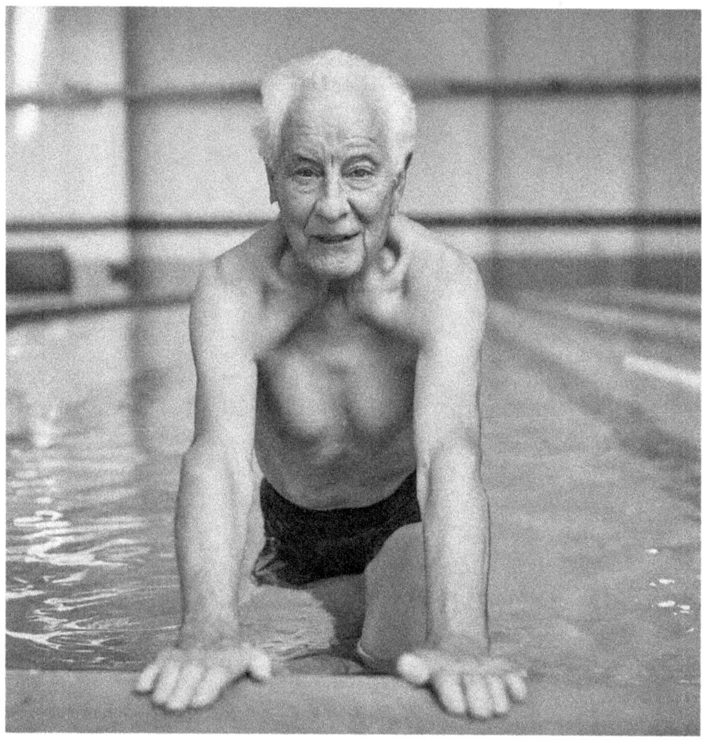

The pendulum leg swings are yet another great workout that can help strengthen your leg, glutes, and abdominal muscles. It is also easy enough to perform that people of all ages can do it.

Here is how to perform this exercise:

- Start by standing at the edge of the pool, in chest-high water.

- While slightly leaning on your right side, lift your left leg a bit. You can even hold onto the edge of the pool to stabilize and balance yourself.

- Slowly swing your left leg forward as much as you can, before pushing it back again as far as you can.

- Continue swinging your leg back and forth while keeping your back and torso straight throughout the exercise.

- Make sure your body is still and that only your legs are moving.

- Continue swinging the leg for 15 to 20 reps before switching to the other leg.

- Repeat the same procedure with the other leg as well and do the same number of sets as your right leg.

39: Karaoke

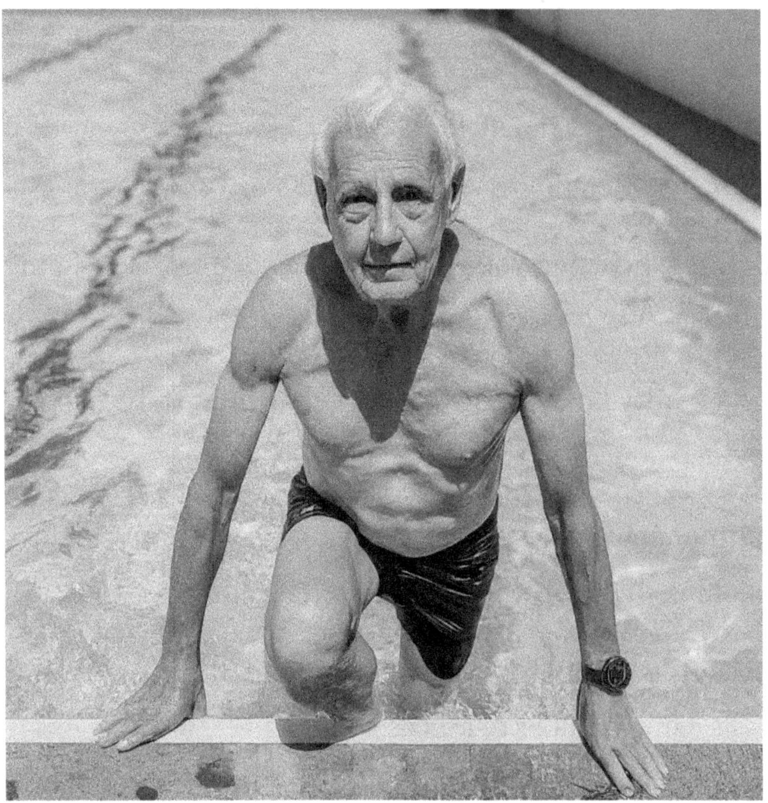

The karaoke exercise is a great workout routine that targets and strengthens your leg and core muscles. It is also easy and fun to perform, making it suitable for all ages, even seniors. This exercise will also put your stability to the test, making you more balanced and strong.

Here is how to perform this exercise:

● Start by standing in a pool of chest-high water.

- To make the exercise more impactful, you can run back and forth across the pool to increase the resistance.

- While standing upright on one edge of the pool, cross your right foot over and in front of your left foot and extend your arms to your side.

- Bring your left foot to your side, then cross your right foot behind your left foot.

- Continue with the same movement laterally then repeat moving in the other direction.

40: Pool running

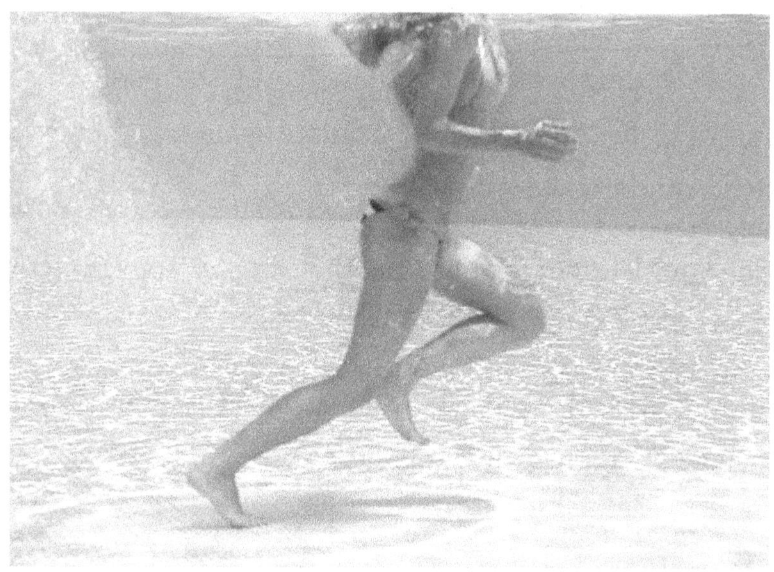

While water jogging is great, pool running is even better because it strengthens your whole body, including your cardiovascular muscles. It is also relatively easy because it is similar to regular running on land. The difference is that jogging in water is more effective because it offers more resistance.

Here is how to do this exercise:

- Start by standing at the edge of the pool, in chest-high water.

- Now start running in a straight line from one edge of the pool to the other side of the pool.

- You can even incorporate butt kicks and high knees to make the exercise more impactful.

- You can also add some flutter kicks once you reach the edge of the pool to make the exercise more effective.

41: Noodle squat

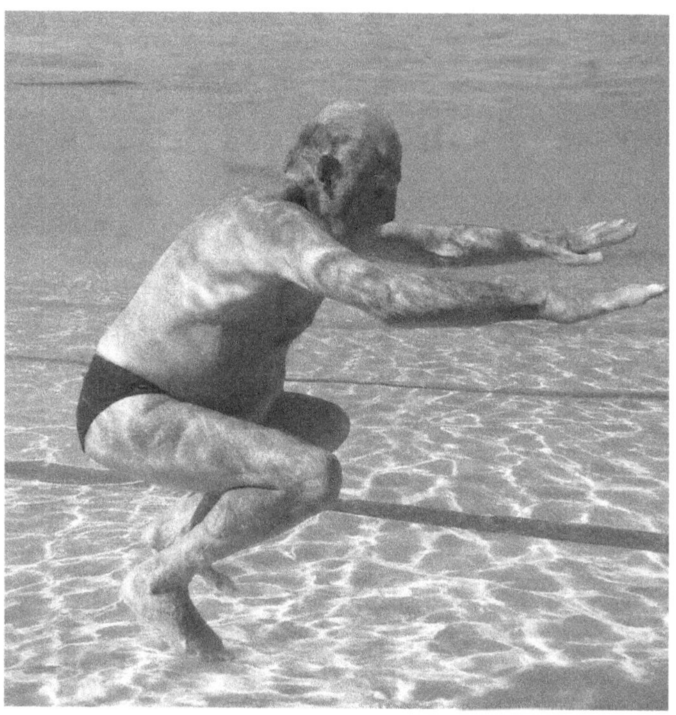

A variation to the normal squats, the noodle squat is a great exercise that strengthens your glutes, leg, and core muscles all at once. Moreover, just like standard squats, noodle squats are easy to perform, making them great for people of all ages, especially seniors. To engage in this exercise, you will need a set of quality noodles.

Here is how to do this exercise:

- Begin by standing in waist-high water.

- Spread your feet shoulder-width apart.

- Place the noodle on the surface of the water in front of you.

- Extend your arms straight and hold the noodle firmly.

- Gradually bend your knees and lower your body into the water.

- Push the noodle down into the water to reach your knees.

- Once you are as low as possible, return to your original position.

- During the squat, sure your back is straight, and your head is above the water.

- Continue with the same procedure for about 15 reps.

42: Calf raises

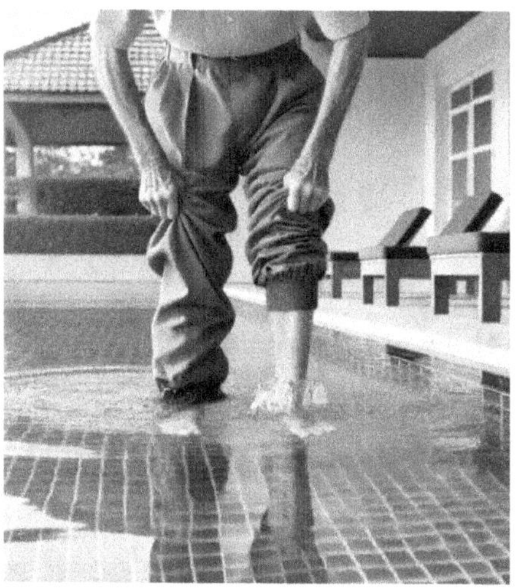

Calf raises strengthen your calves and lower body. It is also a friendly workout routine that is very easy to perform.

Here is how to execute this exercise:

- Start by standing in waist-high water, close to the edge of the swimming pool.

- Stand in an upright position, with your legs together and your arms by your side.

- Now shift your body forward until you stand on your toes.

- Remain in that position for a few seconds before going back to your original position.

- Continue repeating the same procedure for about 15 reps.

Advanced Work Out Exercises

This section contains exercises that are a bit advanced because of the strenuous movements and the equipment involved.

43: Push and pulls

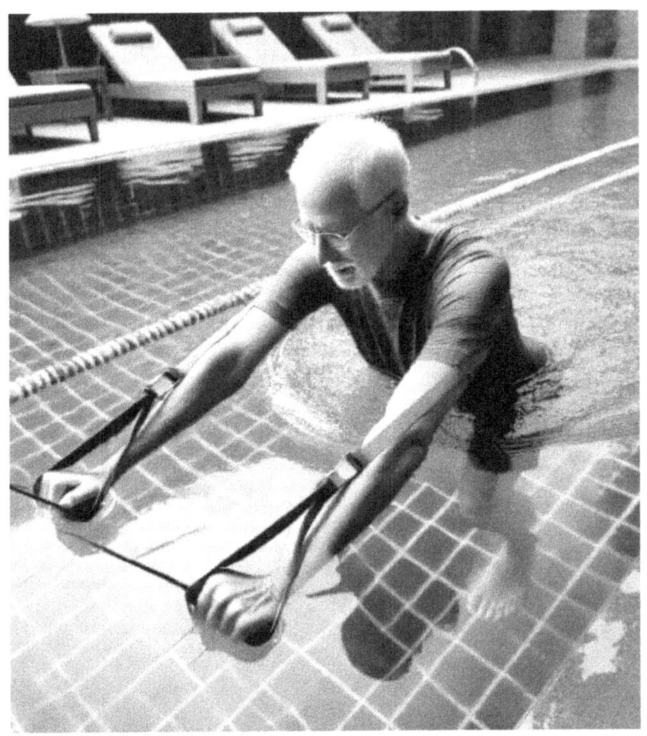

If you'd like to strengthen your arms and core at the same time, then push and pulls is a great workout routine. Compared to other exercises, this exercise is a bit technical, but it is quite effective. The routine requires two dumbbells for extra resistance.

Here is how to do this exercise:

- Begin by standing in chest-high water, in a tall posture.

- Extend your legs shoulder-width apart.

- While holding the dumbbells in each hand, extend both of them slowly until your arms are as straight as possible, then pull your arms back towards your body.

- Make sure you keep the dumbbells below the water surface and that your arms move in a smooth, controlled motion, with your arms swaying your body.

- Additionally, make sure you keep your back straight to avoid injuries.

- Keep repeating the same procedure for ten reps.

44: Side leg raises

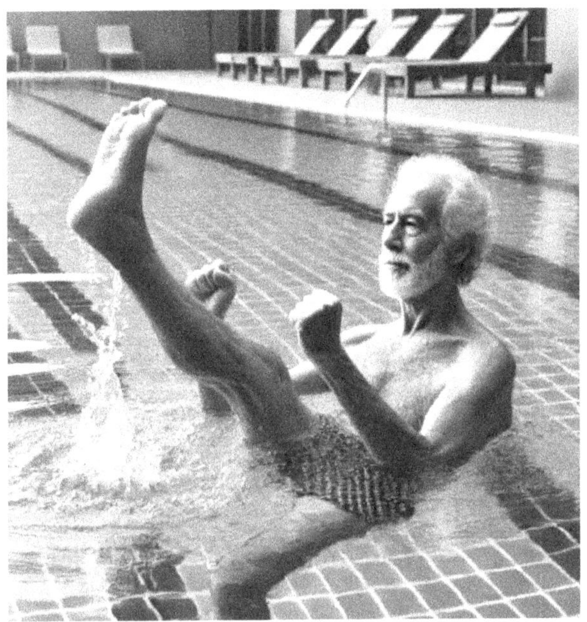

Side leg raises are an advanced water aerobics exercise because, compared to other exercises, this exercise requires you to put in some extra force. However, it is quite effective for strengthening your torso, arm, and leg muscles, all at the same time. You are going to require dumbbells for this exercise—they help you maintain your balance should you lose it while working out.

Here is how to execute it:

- While standing in chest-high water, maintain an upright posture with your feet together.

- Take the dumbbells in each hand on the surface of the water, making sure your keep your arms fully extended out to your sides.

- Lift both dumbbells as high as you can on each side.

- Raise your left leg out to your side by 30 to 45 degrees before returning to your original position.

- Repeat the same procedure then change to the other leg.

- Continue doing this for 10 to 15 reps on each side.

45: *Noodle lifts*

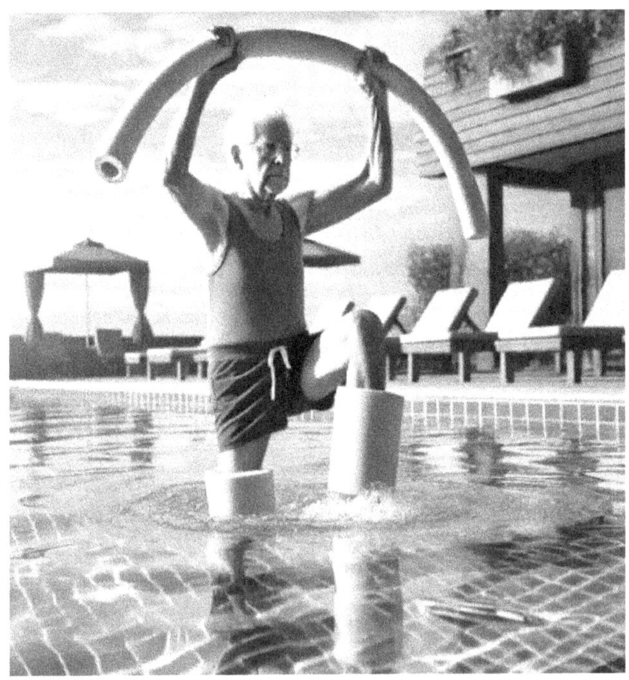

The noodle lifts are a great exercise that you can use to strengthen your chest and arm muscles. The exercise routine is also relatively easy to execute because it does not entail strenuous movements. For this exercise, you will need a noodle.

Here is how to execute it:

- Start by standing in chest-high water, with your feet spread out shoulder-width apart.

- Now hold the noodle in front of your body, with your arms fully extended on the surface of the water.

- Gradually lift the noodle above your head while keeping both your elbows straight then hold that position for 20 seconds.

- Lower the noodle back to the original position then repeat the same procedure.

- Continue for 15 reps, while increasing the speed of each rep.

46: Weighted calf raises

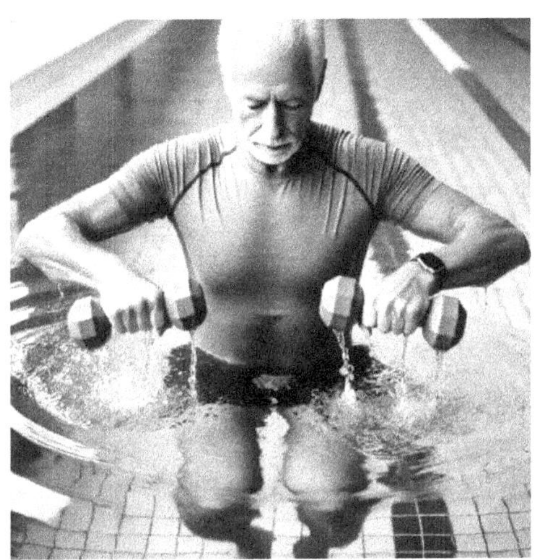

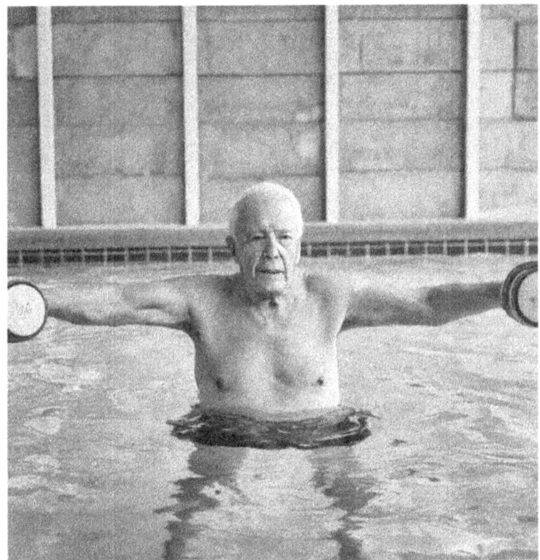

Another great variation of the calf raises we discussed earlier is the weighted calf raises. This exercise is great and better because it offers more resistance than the normal calf raises.

Weighted calf raises help strengthens your leg and arm muscles. It is a more advanced and technical form of water aerobics exercises that you can try if you are looking for great results fast. The exercise requires dumbbells—they help you with stability and recovery should you lose your rhythm while exercising.

Here is how you execute this exercise:

- Begin by standing in chest-high water, with water ankles and your feet together.

- Hold dumbbells, with your arms extended in front of you as much as you can.

- Slowly lift the heels of both feet at the same time to raise your feet off the pool floor.

- Now slowly lower your feet down again, then repeat.

- Continue the same procedure for 10-15 reps.

47: Dumbbells jumping jacks

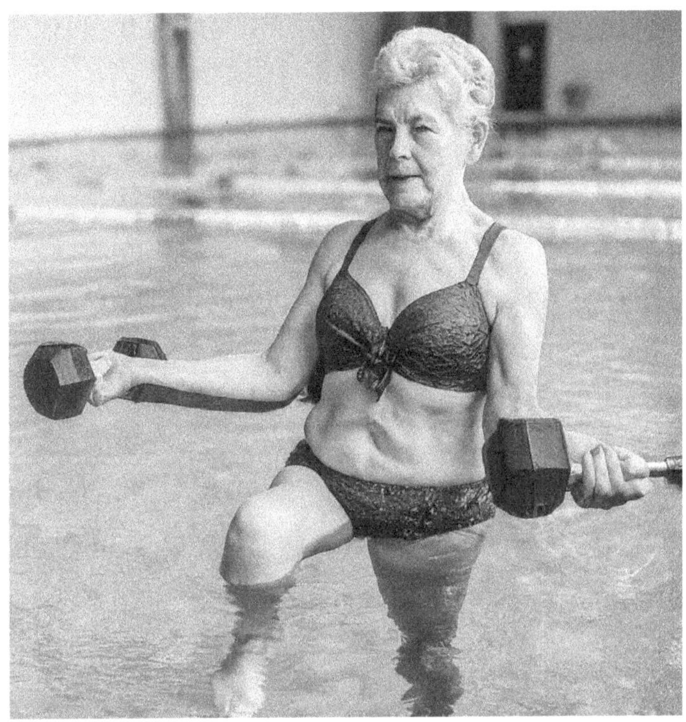

The dumbells jumping jacks are a more advanced version of the jumping jacks; they offer more resistance. This exercise helps strengthen your arms, legs, and core muscles.

The exercise is more advanced than the other kinds of water aerobics exercises, but it also has more pronounced benefits. You are going to need dumbbells for this exercise.

Here is how you can perform this exercise:

- While standing in chest-high water, maintain an upright posture, and keep your feet together.

- Hold the dumbbells against the sides of your body and push your hands into the water.

- Once your arms reach your sides, jump and extend both legs outwards, then lift both your arms outwards at the same time.

- Make sure the dumbbells remain submerged under the water throughout the exercise. Just make sure to lift your arms as high as possible.

- Repeat the procedure for 10-15 reps.

48: Dumbbell torso twists

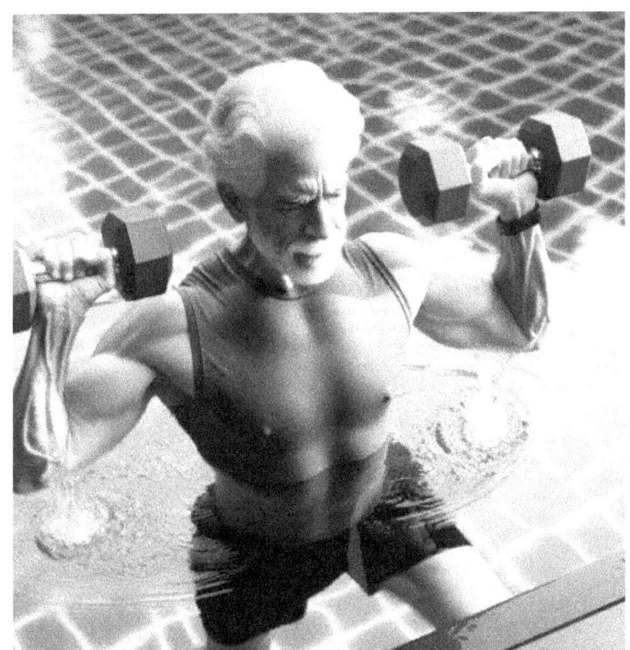

Another technical form of water aerobic is the dumbbell torso twists that strengthens your core and arm muscles. This is an excellent kind of water aerobics that you can try if you are looking to move to the next level of fitness. For this exercise, you are going to need dumbells.

Here is how you execute this exercise.

- Begin by standing in chest-high water, with your legs shoulder-width apart.

- Hold the dumbbells in each hand, then bend your knees to lower your body into a shallow squat.

- Slowly rotate your torso to one side while keeping your arms extended so that the dumbells can move to the same side of your body.

- Repeat the same procedure with your opposite side, then continue with the workout as you alternate sides.

- Do the exercise for ten reps.

50: Sprints

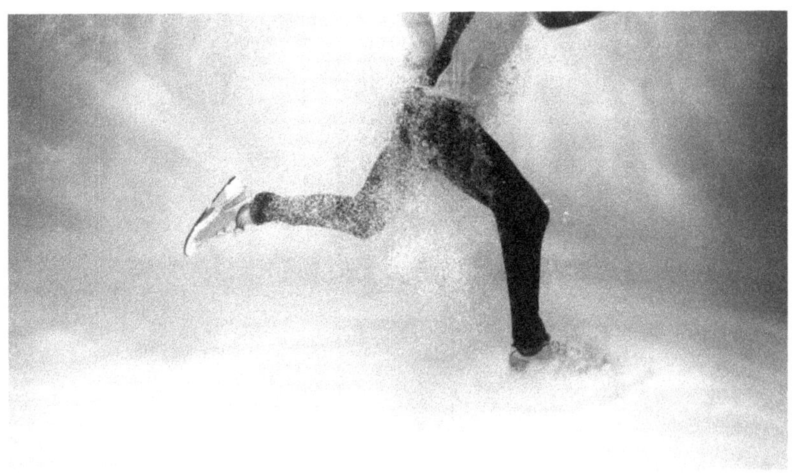

This workout routine is great if you'd like to strengthen your leg muscles and your lower abdomen. It does not require any strenuous movements, which makes it is suitable for all ages, even seniors.

Here is how to execute this exercise:

- Begin by standing in waist-high water, at the edge of the pool.

- Use both arms to hold onto the side of the pool while you maintain an upright posture.

- Keep your legs together.

- Now quickly lift both your legs at the same time to hit your bottom or to reach the surface of the water.

- Return to your original position then repeat the procedure.

- Continue with the movements for 10-15 times.

50: ViPR press and clean

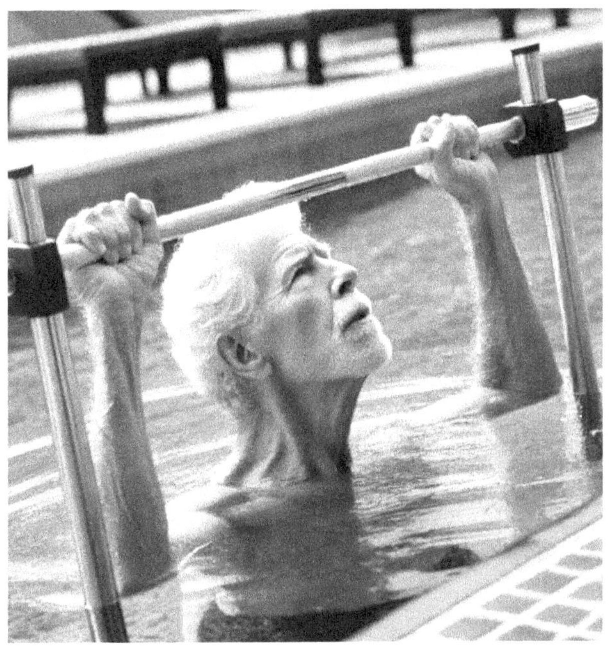

This advanced water aerobics exercise is perfect if you are looking to strengthen your whole body. It may be a bit more advanced than the other aerobics exercises we have discussed, but anyone, even seniors, can perform it with ease. The exercise requires that you have ViPR.

Here is how to perform this exercise:

- Start by standing in chest-high water.

- Hold the ViPR in a way that leaves your hands evenly spaced in the middle.

- Now inhale, then immediately press the ViPR into the water as much as you can while submerging your head.

- Remain in that position for about 20 seconds.

- Gradually lift the ViPR back to the surface then press it over your head.

- Repeat the process for ten reps.

51: Push plate rotation

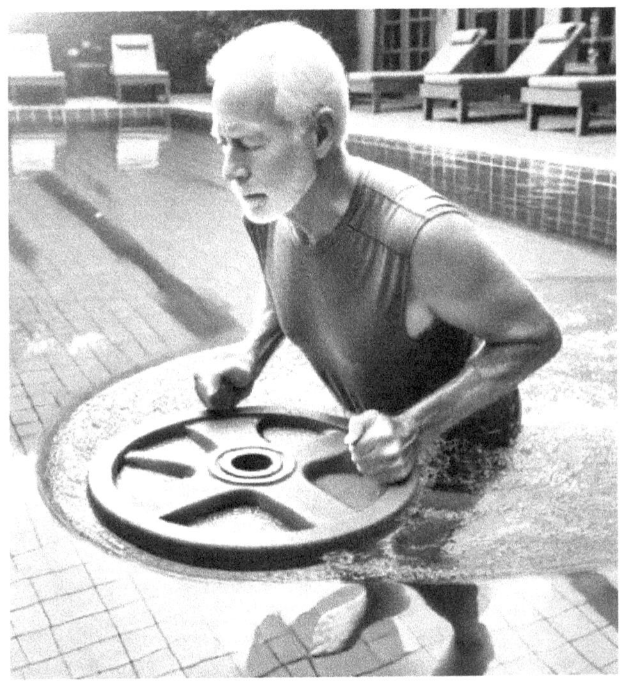

The push plate rotation exercise is also an advanced form of water aerobics that works out and strengthens your arms and core. To perform this exercise, you need a set of push plates—the push plates offer more resistance.

Here is how you perform this exercise:

NOTE: There are two ways to do this exercise. For a less exerting routine, hold the push plate with the yellow blade facing you. If you're looking for a challenging version, hold the push plates by the other side such that the yellow blade is parallel to your arms.

- Start by standing in chest-high water.

- Extend your feet wider than shoulder-width apart, with your knees slightly bent.

- Extend your arms directly in front of your arms, and hold the push plates slightly submerged in the water.

- Tighten your abdominal muscles and rotate your torso from side to side, pushing and pulling the push plates through the water.

- Continue with these movements for 10-15 reps.

52: The Kettlebell swing

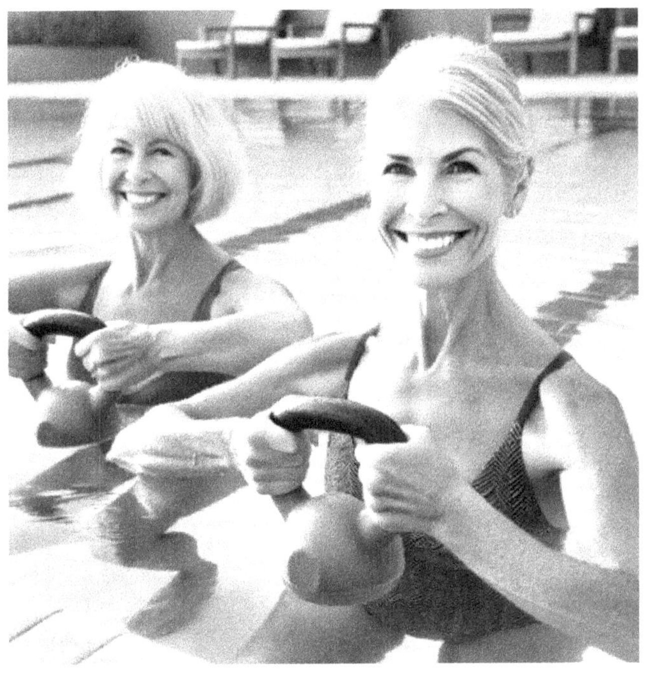

The kettlebell swing is another advanced form of water aerobics exercises that works out and strengthens your posterior chain muscles. To perform this exercise, you will need a heavy kettlebell. The exercise might be a bit strenuous than the other kinds of water aerobics exercises we have discussed, but the results will be worth it.

Here is how to execute this exercise.

- Start by standing in chest-high water.

- Extend your feet shoulder-width apart and bend your knees slightly for a strong foundation.

- Swing the kettlebell by hinging at your hips, and, swinging through your legs, driving it forward, and lift it over your head.

- Allow the kettlebell to swing back down.

- Continue the same procedure for a desired number of reps.

53: Clutch paddles biceps curl

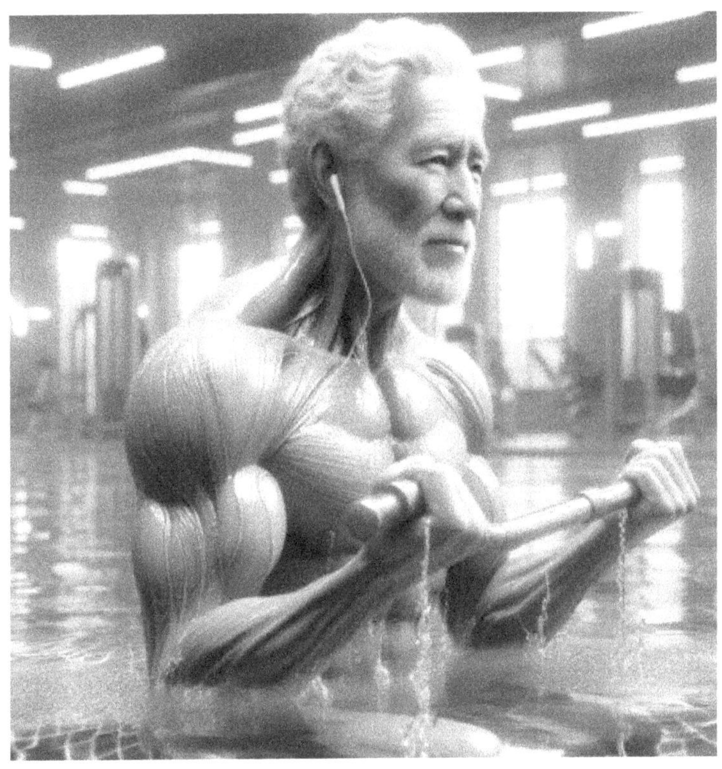

If you are looking for a more advanced workout routine that will help strengthen your biceps and triceps fast, then the clutch paddles biceps curl is the perfect exercise. It might be a bit advanced, but the benefits you stand to gain are many. To perform this exercise, you will need a pair of clutch paddles.

Here is how to execute this exercise:

- Start by standing in chest-high water.

- Affix the clutch paddles to both your arms by fitting the designated rubber tubing around your middle finger and your wrist and place your thumb in the thumb hole.

- Now spread your legs at shoulder-width apart to assume the athletic position.

- Hold the paddles facing away from you and perform biceps curls while keeping the clutch paddles facing up to create as much resistance as possible.

- Once you are at the top of the curl, rotate your wrists such that the paddles face down for extra resistance.

- Press the paddles down to work your triceps then immediately resume into the curl.

- Continue the procedure for ten reps.

54: Jumping jack with push plates

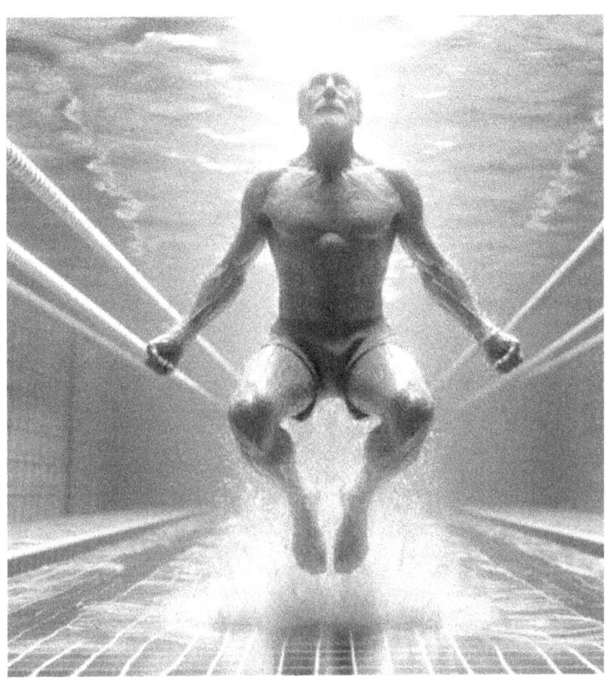

A variation to the standard jumping jacks is to add push plates for extra resistance. This workout routine strengthens your lower body as well as your arm muscles. It is a more advanced water aerobics exercise that yields great results. To execute this routine, you will need push plates.

Here is what you need to do to perform this exercise.

- Begin by standing in chest-high water.

- Now grasp the push plates, with both your arms in front of your torso, extended, and your elbows slightly bent.

- Now bend your knees slightly and lower your body into the water and assume a squat.

- Inhale, then immediately jump up as high as you can.

- Slowly go back into your original position, submerging your head into the water, and getting into a squat.

- Repeat the procedure for 10 to 15 reps.

55: Push plate chest press

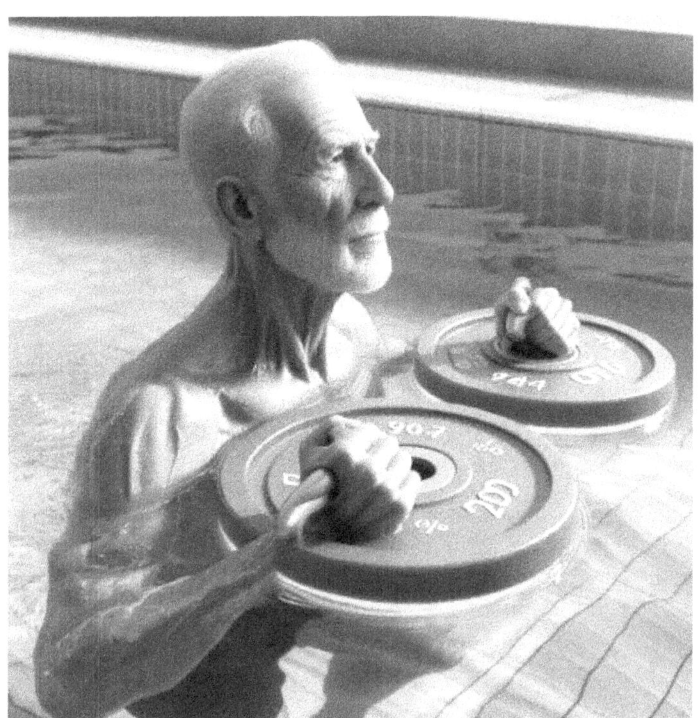

The push plate exercise strengthens your arm and core muscles. The exercise is advanced because it entails some strenuous movements, but people of all ages can perform it. To perform this exercise, you will need push plates.

Here is how to do it:

- Start by standing in chest-high water.

- Hold the push plate by its handle grip on both sides such that the flat side of the plate faces you.

- Bend your knees into a slight squat to assume an athletic stance.

- Submerge the push plate into the water.

- Press the push plate from your chest with powerful, rapid movements, pulling and pushing it through the water.

- Continue these movements for 10 to 15 reps.

Conclusion

If you take action, what you have learned in this guide can help improve your health and strength very rapidly with minimal impact on your joints.

Good luck!

PS: I'd like your feedback. If you are happy with this book, please leave a review on Amazon.

Please leave a review for this book on Amazon by visiting the page below:

https://amzn.to/2VMR5qr